DATE DUE

MR 11 '97			
JA 20 '98			
JY 13 '99			
JE 8 '05			
NO 29 05			
DE 17 05			
DE - 1 '09			

DEMCO 38-296

Lost Lullaby

Lost Lullaby

Deborah Golden Alecson

UNIVERSITY OF CALIFORNIA PRESS
BERKELEY LOS ANGELES LONDON

University of California Press
Berkeley and Los Angeles, California

University of California Press, Ltd.
London, England

© 1995 by the Regents of the University of California

Library of Congress Cataloging-in-Publication Data

Alecson, Deborah Golden, 1954–
Lost lullaby / Deborah Golden Alecson.
     p.   cm.   Includes bibliographical references.
  ISBN 0-520-08870-0 (alk. paper)
  1. Neonatal intensive care—Moral and ethical aspects.
2. Euthanasia—Moral and ethical aspects.   I. Title.
RJ253.5.A44   1995
174'.24—dc20   94-11712
                                                            CIP

Printed in the United States of America
9 8 7 6 5 4 3 2 1
The paper used in this publication meets the minimum
requirements of American National Standard for
Information Sciences—Permanence of Paper for Printed
Library Materials, ANSI Z39.48-1984.

To Lowell, my dearest

I am grateful for your strength and love during the months of Andrea's life, and for your help and support in telling her story.

Contents

Foreword

Having a baby has always carried a potential for tragedy. Mothers can die in labor and delivery, and infants, too, can die, or enter the world with devastating abnormalities, or suffer major trauma during birth. Parental hopes and expectations can be shattered in an instant, leaving a sense of unutterable loss.

Modern obstetric and neonatal care substantially reduces these risks, providing sophisticated technological support for pregnant women and imperiled newborns. Yet, ironically, such care has itself introduced new elements of tragedy.

First, even the best perinatal care falls short of perfection. Deaths still occur, and some neonatal conditions remain irremediable. For parents who have placed unquestioning trust in the power of modern technology, these results carry a cruel taste of disappointment in addition to such natural reactions as grief, anger, and disbelief.

Second, the ability to support but not cure a seriously ill or catastrophically impaired newborn poses extremely disturbing questions about the meaning of leading a human life, the purpose of medical intervention, and the extent of parents' and society's responsibility to provide treatment. These questions have been actively debated for several decades. Health professionals, lawyers, theologians, and ethicists have offered arguments for positions ranging from active euthanasia for any child not able to enter into normal interpersonal interactions to continuing ventilator support for children who meet societally approved definitions of brain death.

Decisions about how much and what kind of treatment to provide for infants with very low odds for survival, or with the potential to survive but with major disabilities, can create tragedy. They highlight the human choices—and the all too human motivations for these choices—that enter into any deliberate action on behalf of another.

Most tragic of all, however, has been the pain and alienation experienced by parents who feel excluded, not only from the normal processes of caring for and nurturing their infants, but also from the decisions that will determine their own and their children's futures. With rare exceptions, parents' voices have been absent, both at the level of national policymaking and in the day-to-day activities of newborn and pediatric intensive care units across the country.

Breaking through this silence, which many parents insist is imposed and not chosen, can itself be painful. No one is certain just how to take into account and respond to parental wishes, requests, suggestions, and demands. Parents do not own their children, but they do share their lives and their stories. What is absolutely clear is that parental silence about care for seriously ill and impaired newborns is ending. Andrea's story is being told, and we must hear it.

Kathleen Nolan, M.D., M.S.L.
Mt. Tremper, NY

Acknowledgments

In writing *Lost Lullaby*, I did not want to rely solely on my own memory and journal notes, so I spoke with many of the other people who were involved. Foremost, I thank the attending neonatologist, whom I've called "Dr. Kravitz" in this book, and Andrea's primary nurse, "Gloria," for taking time away from their demanding jobs to talk with me. Both were generous not only with their memories, but also with their insights into the ethical and medical aspects of neonatology, which are based on perspectives that only they could have.

Over the months, I made many phone calls to gather the recollections of Andrea's original pediatrician "Dr. Minsky," our "guardian angel" "Nancy Cronin," Dr. Kathleen Nolan, "Dr. Maslin," Rose Gasner, "Ricky Pagan," "Joel Damsky," "Dr. Melner," "Dr. Hines," and the friends and family members who had the courage to step into our world at that time. Everyone was more than willing to aid us in reconstructing the past.

Kathy Nolan was an outstanding help to us during Andrea's brief life, and again during the writing of this book. Together we brainstormed the title *Lost Lullaby* (derived from a Jacques Brel song).

I give special thanks to Heide Lange, who worked as my

literary agent. Ms. Lange believed in the importance of the book and, before I did, in my ability as a writer equal to the task. It was her enthusiasm that kept me writing, despite the glorious rejections I received from trade publishers.

Every so often I stumbled upon a medical term or condition that needed clarification. I thank Dr. Michelle Alotta and Dr. Ludwig Klein for answering my questions. Neither of them were directly involved with Andrea, but they supported the writing of this book.

It has been a pleasure having the University of California Press publish the book. Every person involved has been wonderful. I especially pay tribute to Naomi Schneider, the executive editor, who first read the manuscript and expressed a desire to take it on. She made the long-distance, coast-to-coast gap seem inconsequential. I appreciate the prudent attention Tony Hicks gave to the manuscript and Anne Canright's excellent and sensitive editing.

Finally, I honor my mother, Marcia Golden, for having lived through the time of Andrea always present to her emotions and always there for me. Thank you for reading and commenting on the chapters as they unfolded; I know it wasn't easy.

And Lowell: we did more than survive, we evolved.

1

A Perfect Pregnancy

Like every couple that wants to have a child, we hoped for a healthy baby whom we would watch unfold over the months and years into a delightful person in love with the world.

When I found myself pregnant after several months of trying, we had no reason to believe that our hope would not come true. We had weathered a miscarriage earlier on, cause unknown and of no obstetric concern, and so were prepared to feel somewhat anxious until we passed the thirteenth week of this new pregnancy. But aside from that, we had no cause to feel that after nine months of normal gestation, a mystical newborn would not emerge from the cushion of my womb into the cushion of our arms.

When I was growing up I never imagined getting married, let alone having children. The nuclear family into which I was born had already disintegrated by the time I was a toddler. I was wary of that institution, as I was of many traditional goals in society. I planned to be a free spirit, making my life up as I went along. This feeling altered

forever when I met Lowell. For the first time I loved someone enough to make a lifelong commitment. My adoration
and respect for him helped me to understand the sense and
sanctity of marriage. And then, after a couple of years with
him, I also came to understand why people have children.
Our child would be an extension of the love our union
created.

Our living situation was comfortable for the two of us, but
hardly ideal for the raising of a child, dwelling as we were
in a fourth-floor walk-up apartment.

When I told my father the news of the pregnancy, he
followed his congratulations with, "Of course you'll have to
move. Where will you put the baby?"

"After all, Dad, how much space does an infant take up?"
I replied. The apartment was small, but we were certain that
with some rearranging of furniture a cozy corner could be
created to fit a crib and changing table. I was enthralled
with my pregnant state. Lowell asked, "What does it feel
like?"

"My breasts ache and my nipples are galvanized, like
they're antennae picking up signals from the great
beyond." He listened to my descriptions of a body possessed, but what I was going through was a phenomenon
that nature intended for women only. As I transformed
with the life inside of me, Lowell's thoughts turned to his
role as provider. He worked as a choral director in a sub-
urban high school and gave singing lessons at home. His
concerns were, "Are we going to be able to manage on my
salary alone? How long are you going to stay home with
the baby?" We agreed that I should nurse for as long as I
could, that it would be healthier for the baby and for me. I
wanted to be a full-time mommy for at least the first three
years, if we could afford it.

We wasted no time before broadcasting our good fortune

to our families and friends. After I told my mother, who was thrilled, I called Rhonda, my closest buddy from the high school where I had taught in the special education department. "Rhonda, I'm pregnant. It must have been the time I stood on my head."

"Hooray for you and Lowell! See, I knew it wouldn't take long. Do you have a doctor?"

"No, not yet. I think I'm going to check out midwifery programs."

"You're not going to use midwives!" she exclaimed. She had had complications with the birth of her one-and-a-half-year-old daughter and was emphatic that one should always use an obstetrician. She was convinced that her doctor had saved not only her baby's life, but hers as well. "Deborah, anything could happen. Women have died in childbirth. If something should go wrong. . . . Please, do me a favor and use a doctor." "I'll talk to Lowell," I said, and changed the subject.

My father made jokes about Lowell's astonishing virility, for I had become pregnant both times soon after trying. My mother-in-law wished us well in her way, which also included apprehension: "Oh, we're so happy for you and we just hope everything goes okay this time."

In my second month, morning sickness struck and I staggered through the days. I carried crushed crackers in plastic bags wherever I went, and when lecturing my students at the college I would often need to stop in mid-sentence to ingest a few pieces. My digestion was so out of whack that a food as bland as plain yogurt caused the heartburn of a meatball wedge.

When I wasn't seized by exhaustion or indigestion, I was overcome by the wonder of it all. Not a second went by when I wasn't aware of being pregnant, and each new day I experienced the diminishing importance of previous obsessions and concerns. However, a pressing decision had to be made: the choice of practitioner to deliver the baby.

After some consideration, and despite Rhonda's warning, I decided that I wanted to use a midwife, and that the baby should be born in a hospital. Lowell had reservations.

I explained, "Why should we pay an obstetrician four thousand dollars when we could pay a midwife half that and, most important, be the ones in control?" He responded, "You want to use a midwife after what happened with the miscarriage?"

With the first pregnancy, we were going to use a birthing room in a midwifery practice. When I started to bleed heavily near the end of the first trimester, I ended up in the emergency room of the Catholic hospital that the midwives used as a contingency facility. For over twelve hours I was left to bleed and labor until the obstetrician on call (the backup doctor for the backup doctor for the midwives) was firmly convinced that the embryo was nonviable and that he could perform a D & C without violating the institution's stance on abortion.

"Lowell, it's true that that was a nightmare, but this time we'll be in a hospital from the beginning, so if anything should go wrong . . ." I tried to brush his worry aside. I simply felt that I would be more comfortable with midwives, whereas doctors, whom I distrusted, would orchestrate the birth of my baby for their convenience. I suspected obstetricians of discouraging vaginal births and encouraging Caesarean sections not only so they could charge more money, but also to hasten the process so they could make it to the golf course before sundown. "Midwives," I told Lowell, "will let me labor for as long as I have to in as many ways as I have to. I'll be more relaxed with them."

As fate would have it, a hospital within walking distance of our apartment had a midwifery program. When I called their office (at a separate location), I was told to visit the hospital first and get a tour from one of the midwives. The tour revealed labor and birthing rooms painted a gray-green more appropriate to the interior of a factory, completely lacking in femininity or domesticity. These were rooms where you went to take care of business, and then you left. I was disappointed. Our guide, Lucy, was a large, jovial woman, one of the three midwives in the practice. She promoted the program without being aggressive, inviting us to use it if we were relatively low risk. On leaving the hospital, I turned to one of the other pregnant women on the tour and asked if she had heard good things about the practice.

It turned out she was British, and she answered, "I would only use midwives. My first child, in England, was born naturally with a midwife. I'm definitely going to use them, since I live just down the street."

Her endorsement, the convenience of the location, and the price convinced me.

When I was in my eighth week, Lowell and I had our first appointment with the midwives at their location. Their office had an atmosphere more to my liking. It was painted in pastel shades with flowered boxes of tissues, plants placed just so, and Georgia O'Keeffe–ish prints adorning the walls. Lowell and I sat side by side on the couch, leafing through the parenting magazines that were heaped on the end tables, feeling as if we were being initiated into a new culture. As we waited to see Margaret (one of the midwives) for my first exam, we silently absorbed the reality of our situation.

We were led into one of several immaculate examining rooms, which contained the essentials of obstetrics arranged for maximum efficiency in a small space. Lowell's presence increased my sense that although I was the one in whom our baby was growing, it was our pregnancy, a joint venture. Margaret was pleasant and reassuring, having nothing negative to report except for a lump she found in my expanding right breast. When the exam was over I asked, "So, I'm really pregnant?" and she assured me that I was. Lowell and I walked out of the center feeling good and wise about our choice of practitioners, though our exuberance was slightly marred by the discovery of the lump.

After two months, morning sickness abated, energy returned, and the lump was found to be innocuous. My waistline was replaced with a rounding belly, making me look pudgy, not pregnant. Rhonda called to say she'd stop by with her husband to deliver the "baby stuff" she had been saving. Lowell and I cleared a little space in our one and only closet. Up four flights of stairs and into our apartment they carried five heavy-duty garbage bags bursting with burp cloths, teeny-weeny shoes and socks, plastic pants, stretchies, hats, carriers for the front and carriers for the back, rattles, balls, doodads whose use and purpose we could not fathom but that were, we were assured, necessary—and on and on and on. We kept exclaiming, "Oh my God, oh my God, *look* at all these things!"

Rhonda, envisioning our child, picked out a red velveteen dress with white ruffled sleeves and said, "This will look great with her golden curls." As a child, I had had waves of golden hair. "When I was pregnant with Tessa," Rhonda explained, "I used to keep the clothes I had for her in a dresser, and I'd pull them out just to sniff them."

Lowell, seeing that there wasn't any room left for us to sit and talk, said, "Why don't we move into the other room?" but they had to leave. As we embraced I said thank you over and over again. I noticed Rhonda's sigh of relief as she walked out the door. She had finally gotten rid of those things that took up so much space.

After they left, I began to empty the bags with a crazy abandon. I noticed an aroma, an Ivory Snow scent that sweetened the air. Lowell selected a T-shirt that was stained—with regurgitated breast milk, no doubt—and asked, "What does '1 T' mean?"

"I have no idea. I can't tell what fits a newborn and what fits a six-month-old," I answered, a touch hysterically.

As I plunged into the bags, I observed a growing agitation in Lowell's behavior. "Where are we going to keep all of this?" he asked. I tried to begin sorting things, but I didn't have a system. It was an avalanche. There were boys' clothes and girls' clothes everywhere, and finally I just had to leave the chaos as it was, with attempted piles of seemingly similar things on the floor, couch, chairs, TV, bookshelves, and piano, and go to bed. There was a slight tension between Lowell and me, and I fell asleep feeling as if I had been buried alive.

I had an amniocentesis and ultrasound before Christmas, which meant having to wait a bit longer for the results because of the holidays. The first part was astounding. The sonogram revealed a perfectly developed fetus whose limbs flexed and whose body tumbled. Searching between the legs we were able to conclude that a girl was in the making. I lay on the table, holding Lowell's hand, as a technician rolled the scanner in its cool gel along my abdomen. We were in tears. It was by far the most profound verification—an emotional witnessing—that reproduction was indeed taking place. Here it was, in black and white, a squirming creation that would one day be our daughter.

The second part caused both of us physical discomfort. The insertion of the hollow needle through my abdominal wall was done by Dr. Kembel, the midwives' obstetrician. A dour man of few words, he hurried into the examining room and, with little eye contact or explanation of the procedure, prepared my belly for the needle. As he thrust it through my skin, Lowell, watching nearby, became sick to his stomach, started to faint, and had to be seated by the nurse. To our horror, Kembel missed the amniotic sac and had to do it again, this time successfully.

As he left the room I called to him, "When can we expect the results?"

"After the New Year," he replied, heading down the hallway.

I said to myself, "This man reminds me of why I want midwives."

By January I was fully aware of the presence gyrating inside me. I named this spinning top Lacey. Once the movements were felt, that amorphous being became my potential child. Seeing the fetus on a screen and learning of the sex generated a relationship in my mind. I believe that human life begins at birth and not at conception, so Lacey's personhood at five months' gestation did not seem real to me. And yet I thought of her and referred to her as something, if not yet a person. I was bonding with her, whatever she was. I began to function as a "we" instead of an "I," conscious always of how the world was affecting both of us.

My sixth month began with the blessed news that the amniocentesis results were normal. I wrote in my journal:

> Lacey's presence is ever known. I can feel her moving just about all the time. Last night Lowell witnessed her thrusts through my belly. I would like to think her strong activity indicates her strength and health. I was extremely affected by the Baka people as shown on that National Geographic film. First of all, they all seemed so happy and peaceful. I was impressed by the mother, nine months pregnant, hand-fishing in the river and building a clay dam. When she felt it was time to give birth she calmly told her husband, who rubbed estrogen plant extract on her belly. During the night, with no need of anyone besides her husband, she gave birth. And in the morning,

while the newborn girl stretched and felt life, Momma's concern was that her youngest son should accept his new sister. She showed no signs of having undergone what I anticipate to be the biggest ordeal in a woman's life. Momma was perfectly present, alert, and at rest. Then again, that was her third child and she was twenty-four years old.

I carried around the image of that Baka woman as my pregnancy became more obvious. I walked the streets of my jittery neighborhood, proud in my maternity, at one with the pregnant women of the world. I was a natural being in an artificial world of concrete, asphalt, and brick. In a bathing suit that resembled a parachute, I'd lower myself into the pool at the club and swim lap after lap, sensing the increased oxygen spreading throughout my body and rushing through Lacey's. I wasn't snatching wiggling fish from a stream, but I was striving for the utmost physicality possible, given my urban environment. I was in a different sort of jungle that required the same degree of alertness. Like the Baka woman, I had to protect my progeny from danger. I walked along the avenues with deliberate steps and darting eyes. I felt a vulnerability such as I had never experienced before. The animals that stampeded in this environment had horns that honked and could run me over.

In my fantasy, like the Baka woman I, too, would squat in the night under the stars and moon and bring forth my child.

At the pool one day I became acquainted with a pregnant woman named Leona. She was expecting a girl at the end of March, and like me she exercised every day regardless of physical ills or an enlarging belly (though hers was small and compact). Leona worked as a nurse in a hospital's neonatal intensive care unit (NICU) and planned to take a maternity leave. Although I understood that she worked with sick babies, I hadn't an inkling of how technical her responsibilities were. There was no reason for me to think that Lacey would need an NICU; after all, as far as I could tell, the babies in Leona's care were premature or born to drug addicts. *Our* babies were destined to be healthy and normal.

"Let's keep in touch," she suggested, "and after our babies are born, we'll take them to the pool and you and I can take turns swimming and watching them."

"That sounds terrific. My biggest concern about the arrival of the baby has been how I'd be able to fit swimming in every day. Let's work something out," I said as we exchanged phone numbers.

I was into the third trimester when, one morning, Lowell said, "Deb, I've been thinking about it, and I want her name to be Andrea. I never liked Lacey, and I want her to be named after my aunt Andrea."

For three months I'd had a Lacey in my belly, so it was difficult to give up that identity. My mother, earlier that week, had taken me aside and with profound gravity said, "Deb, I think you'd be making a big mistake by naming the baby Lacey." I got defensive immediately.

"What's wrong with Lacey? I like that name." My mother, the psychologist, replied, "It's too prissy. It's the name for a docile lamb. It would affect her character. Lacey brings to mind a certain image that I'm sure you don't want your daughter to have."

"Ma, I totally disagree with you." I didn't want to discuss it further.

I had to discuss it with Lowell, though. The name Andrea would embrace both Lowell's aunt and my favorite aunt, Anna, also dead. It was a beautiful and appropriate name for our daughter, and I had to concede. As soon as that was decided, Lowell became extremely animated, talking and singing to Andrea through my belly.

Leona called one morning on a day we were to meet at the pool and later go furniture shopping for the babies. She told me she was in labor. "I'll go to the hospital after I get done doing the laundry," she said.

"I can't believe you're doing a mundane thing like the laundry when you're on the brink of the miraculous. Leona, it must not be bad if you can wash clothes." I was amazed. "Tell me about it. How does it feel?"

"It's no big deal. I have to go now and put the clothes in the dryer."

The next day, bearing flowers, I walked into the maternity ward of the hospital where Leona had given birth (and at which she worked). I met her parents, who were sitting beside her bed beaming away, and embraced the new mother. Alice, who had slipped right out after a brief struggle, was nestled in her arms, nursing. Watching them, I realized with a renewed understanding that this—the baby—is what pregnancy is all about. Pregnancy is not an end in itself. There before me lived and breathed a creature who just hours ago was inside Leona. In a matter of weeks I, too, would come face to face with the creature inside me.

Our first Lamaze class at the hospital was in the evening, at what I considered to be a late hour to venture out but was really a reasonable hour for nonpregnant people. I dressed in my black stretch pants, oversized black-and-red striped T-shirt, and white Keds. "Am I dressed nonchalant?" I asked Lowell, hoping to disguise my nervousness. All I wanted to do was collapse on our couch with my feet up and read until I passed out (my usual after-dinner routine during my pregnancy). I couldn't believe that I would have to be alert for the next two hours.

We sat with seven other couples on padded metal chairs

in the dreary room reserved for natural childbirth classes. Upon entering the room, we had found a stack of magazine articles on each seat, which we automatically started to read, relieved at not having to acknowledge one another. I found being one of eight pregnant women in the same room funny and a little embarrassing. The specialness I had grown to feel was either gone or exaggerated, I couldn't tell which. Each of our private wonders was proved to be commonplace. It was as if we shared a secret that was obvious to all the world. I knew that although the other women appeared mindful of their surroundings, they were in fact, as I was, completely preoccupied with the hiccups and kicks of the fetus and the tingling sensations of their breasts. In my thoughts I was comparing belly sizes, shapes, and positions. "That woman is huge. It can't all be baby. Boy, will she ever be sorry after the baby is born and she has to lose that weight. And that gal with the high heels, how on earth does she maneuver in those?" Here I was athletic and fit, as if pregnancy was some kind of sport you had to train for.

Our instructor, Pamela, having wandered around introducing herself, now began our session. As a registered nurse she knew her facts, but not being a professional teacher she imparted this information in a rambling fashion that, given the hour of the evening, was, I thought, oddly appropriate. The best part was saved for the end of class, when we were all more relaxed. Stretched out on the floor in couples, practically on top of one another in the small room, we concentrated on the style and timing of breaths. The stillness of the air was penetrated by the women's exhalations and inhalations and our husbands' murmurs of encouragement. It was an intimate, almost sexual experience; Lowell and I looked forward to going home to practice.

At the end of April, my mother had a baby shower for me at her apartment in Brooklyn. Leona, with Alice, drove us from Manhattan in her yellow Volkswagen bug. The females of my family and a few friends gathered at my mother's terraced apartment, with views of the beach at Coney Island and the Manhattan skyline, like some Emerald City, in the far distance. I was wearing a pink dress that really emphasized my belly, and my cousin Judy couldn't resist commenting (for she knew how hard I worked to keep in shape), "Hey Deb, what are you carrying? Twins?"

"She doesn't even look pregnant from behind," someone piped up.

My mother prepared a gargantuan spread of bagels, cream cheese, lox, cold cuts, fruit, and apple pie, which we gorged on while I opened presents. There was a baby shower custom that I knew nothing about and that Judy officiated over: the making of a hat out of the ribbons, bows, and wrapping paper, with a new ornament being added as each gift was unwrapped. I received for Andrea the tiniest items, so cute, so sweet, so pink. Everything from the flowered crib sheets to the dresses was a different intensity and shade of pink. When all the gifts were unwrapped, photos were taken of me parked on my mother's couch, laughing with that outlandish hat perched on my head. I felt blessed and excited as I imagined each gift in use. I saw Andrea naked on the changing table kicking her feet as the black-and-white mobile that Leona had given us dangled above her head. I saw her listening to the music box Judy had bought, watching the carousel horse revolve around its shiny brass pole. The occasion of the shower and the sharing with family and friends deepened my faith in how right everything would be.

May arrived at last, with weekly visits to the midwives, the college semester coming to an end, and our last Lamaze classes at the hospital. Something had gone wrong with the pregnancies of everyone in our group, with the sole exception of mine. One woman had developed diabetes; another's baby was in breech position, guaranteeing a Caesarean section; and the youngest woman in the class had gone into premature labor. In class we had talked about a few of the things that could go wrong and about Caesareans, but I hardly paid attention. I was the Baka woman. I was swimming a mile a day in my ninth month. I was so certain of a perfect labor and pregnancy that I had written in my journal:

> God Almighty—Andrea is really and truly on her way. I predict an absolutely normal delivery—average in pain and duration. Margaret said my pelvis is a good size and that the baby is not huge.

May 23, due date. I awoke at five in the morning from a brief, fitful sleep, feeling crampish and ill. I couldn't even imagine dragging myself across the pool.

When Lowell woke up I told him, "Lowell, today's the day. I feel too sick for it not to be. I'm supposed to see the midwives this afternoon, but I'm going to call them now and see if I can get an appointment this morning."

"Should I go to work?" he asked.

"Oh, absolutely. Nothing is going to happen for a while."

At their office, June, one of the three midwives, examined me and found that I was fifty percent effaced with my cervix closed.

She said, "You don't want to go into labor yet. If you go into labor tonight, it will be a long one."

Did I have a choice? I went home and passed the day lying inert on the couch, reading and rereading the sections about labor and birth in my five manuals, pages of text I already knew by heart. It wasn't until the evening, while talking on the phone with Kitty, my stepmother, that I felt a definite contraction.

"Kitty, I just had a contraction. I mean, I think it was one. Let's keep on talking and I'll see what happens."

More contractions followed, and of course I couldn't talk, and Kitty couldn't talk: we were both too excited. "I'd better hang up and time them."

"Call us as soon as you know whether it's the real thing," she said.

Lowell, proving to us both that he had actually paid attention in class and knew what he was doing, timed my contractions. They were sporadic, following no discernible pattern. "Call the midwives and let's see what they think," Lowell said.

Margaret was on duty. After hearing my report, she concluded, "Considering that your cervix was closed this morning, birth is a long ways off. You're ready for the three B's: bath, brandy, and bed. Try to relax and get some sleep."

"Try to relax? Try to sleep? She must be kidding," I said to Lowell when I got off the phone. "Where's the brandy?" I asked, knowing full well where it was, bought months ago for this very occasion.

After my bath and brandy, I joined Lowell in bed. He was already asleep ("One of us should try to get some rest, at least," I'd told him), but it was impossible for me to fall asleep. The contractions were increasing in intensity; they were all I could think about. Finally, at two in the morning, I called the midwives and spoke with Margaret, who said, "When the contractions are five minutes apart you'll be ready to come to the hospital. In the meantime, have more brandy and try to rest."

"Try to rest? There's no way in hell I can rest," I thought, and poured myself two mouthfuls of brandy.

Back in bed, I shifted from one position to another, trying in vain to get comfortable. Lowell, aware of my nocturnal activities, roused himself and offered, "Do you want me to rub your feet?"

"I'd love you to. But first let's time the contractions."

They were getting more regular, but they weren't coming rapidly enough to impress the midwives. I left Lowell in bed after he had lovingly massaged my feet, hoping that he would fall asleep. I realized that I was hungry, so I consumed a bowl of raisin bran cereal, taking spoonfuls between the waves of pain. I held on until ten before calling the midwives. Lucy was on duty.

"You've got to see me. I'm in agony," I pleaded. Lucy granted me permission to come to the hospital, and I immediately alerted Lowell.

We assumed this was it, so we packed my bags with all the accoutrements of natural childbirth, including relaxation tapes and one tape of Lowell singing songs especially for me. By this time I couldn't dress myself, and Lowell had to put on my shoes and comb my hair. I had to brace myself against a wall or Lowell every time a contraction came on.

Lucy's examination showed that I was seventy-five percent effaced but only one to two centimeters dilated.

"I can't believe it," I cried, "all this pain and so little progress. How can this be? Lucy, I don't think I can take it any more. Give me something for the pain."

So much for natural childbirth. "I'll give you three alternatives," Lucy said. She was standing at the foot of my bed after having heard a strong fetal heartbeat from the Doppler. "You can stay at the hospital—but I'm warning you, you'd be here a long time—and get pain medication; you can go home and take pain medication with you; or you can go home without a painkiller. It's up to you."

"What's a long time?" I croaked.

"At least twelve hours."

Lowell gathered up my bags, pillow, tape recorder, and

pregnancy text, and I went home with a couple of Nembu-
tals.

I was already losing sight of the purpose, the meaning of
my agony, which was the birth of our daughter, the ultimate
joy of our lives. I was consumed with stabbing pains that
wouldn't go away, that in fact sharpened with each passing
hour. The Nembutal was undetectable; morphine might
have done the trick.

My mother arrived at two in the afternoon, to be present
at the birth. She found me where I had been for the previous
two hours: in the bathtub.

"Ma, there are no words to describe what I am going
through. I don't know how much more I can take," I
greeted her as she entered the bathroom.

She sat down on the toilet seat beside the tub. "You'll
take as much as you have to take."

I couldn't argue with that. I remained in the bathtub for
another four hours, my skin turning a grayish white, while
Lowell and my mother ate Chinese take-out food in the
nursery. The smell made me gag.

At six P.M., twenty-four hours after I had felt the first
contraction, I was admitted to the hospital. June was the
midwife on duty, and after completing her exam she told
me, "The good news is, you're one hundred percent effaced. The bad news is, you're still only one to two centimeters dilated." Then she strapped an external monitor around
my belly and gave me the shot of Demerol I had begged for.

For the next three and a half hours I lay on my back
writhing in pain, journeying further and further away from
reality, only hazily aware of the comings and goings of Lowell, my mother, June, and the nurses. At nine-thirty, June
made a decision: "I think it would be best to give you
Pitocin. You're not making progress on your own. It will
help get things going."

I had read about Pitocin and vaguely recollected that it could make the contractions more severe. But there was also something else, something having to do with complications.

"I don't think so, June. It will make things worse—if that's possible."

"I assure you," she said, "you won't even notice a difference."

I had been in labor for over twenty-four hours, and I hadn't slept in thirty-six. I had to trust June's judgment. I gave my consent.

Five or six more hours passed. I was given another dose of Pitocin. At one point, when June told me that I was eight to nine centimeters dilated, I tried to push. By now, all propriety, modesty, and grasp of ordinary life had vanished. I was, as I had been for most of the evening, lying on my back. Lowell grabbed one leg and a nurse the other, lifting them high into the air. They offered words of encouragement as I did what I believed to be pushing the baby out. June would cheer, "Come on, come on, you can do it." She even told me that the baby's head was in view. I couldn't tell what was happening. I pushed, I strained, I lost bladder and rectal control as my body trembled uncontrollably from the waist down. But all this effort got us nowhere.

More Demerol, then oxygen. And then a familiar face appeared, that of Dr. Kembel. June, without our knowledge, had gotten him from the next room, where a patient of his was in labor. He briefly acknowledged me as he made a beeline to the fetal monitor. He sat on the edge of the bed by my feet looking intently at the monitor strips, with June standing close by. He pointed to something on the strips, which June, apparently, had spoken to him about. Without saying anything to either Lowell or me, they left the room.

Soon after, Dr. Kembel returned to say, "The baby's not coming down, so we'll have to do a C-section." I was expecting to hear this and was, in fact, relieved. I asked, "Can I have an epidural?"

"No. You'll need general anesthesia." When I asked him why, he gave me an answer that seemed to make sense at the time.

He left the room, and Lowell asked June, "Will I still be able to be present during the birth?"

She replied, "Yes, I don't see why not."

"Can I bring in the camera?" he asked.

"Yes, that's fine."

She handed him a blue paper gown, slippers, mask, and hat and ushered him to a restroom where he could change.

There followed a flurry of activity as papers where brought for me to sign. Then a troop of nurses materialized to move me into the operating room. I developed a massive leg cramp, to which they seemed insensitive as they pulled and tugged me onto the table. I cried out for them to be gentle, but their maneuvering of me felt frantic and rough.

The wave of excitement I felt knowing labor was about to end and that I was finally to have my baby was quickly succeeded by a chill of dread.

In the operating room, as they strapped down my arms and legs—which only increased the terrifying spasm in my leg—and shaved my lower belly and pubic hair, June searched for the fetal heartbeat. She couldn't find it.

"Get another monitor!" I screamed, barely recognizing my own voice.

Again, no heartbeat. A woman I had never seen before inserted an internal monitor through my vagina to attach to the baby's head as I yelled, "Where's the anesthesiologist? What's taking her so long? My leg!" The anesthesiologist soon arrived and, standing behind my head, placed the mask on my face. "It's not on tight enough. The stuff's leaking out the sides . . ." Then I lost consciousness.

Lowell had been left outside the door, ignored by June and Dr. Kembel. He stood in the sanitized blue outfit, listening to the frenzy within and watching as one monitor was wheeled out of the room and another wheeled in.

Then he waited for the cry that did not come.

2

Andrea Is Born

When I regained consciousness in the recovery room, I found my father, stepmother, and Lowell standing at the foot of my bed. They appeared as the shadowy forms of people I knew and loved, but they were not smiling and exclaiming, "Congratulations!" The fact that I wasn't wearing my eyeglasses added to my disorientation. Yet even in my postoperative haze, I knew from their silence that something horrible had happened. This conclusion was quickly followed by denial: No, it can't be; Andrea must be in the nursery, sleeping. I felt an urgent need to hold and nurse her, for I had learned that bonding should be initiated immediately after birth. I also didn't want her to be given the dreaded sugar water when what she needed was colostrum, the elixir of breast milk.

Struggling to transfer my thoughts to my mouth, I slurred the words, "Where's Andrea? I want to nurse her."

It was my father who spoke first, "She's in the nursery, Deb. She's being looked at by the doctors. There was a little trouble . . ."

"She's very sick," Lowell said.

In the blur I saw Lowell's face, and I knew that he had been crying. Then his voice dissolved as I succumbed to sleep.

It wasn't until late morning that I awoke to a certain degree and became semi-cognizant of my surroundings, though I was still confused about my circumstances. Noticing the absence of other women in nearby beds, I deduced that I was in a private room, a luxury we hadn't asked for since our health insurance didn't cover it. I worried that the accommodations were going to cost us a fortune. Needles stuck out of veins in the back of my hand, and I experienced a restricting tightness below my waist. It took several seconds for me to realize that that sensation was coming from my belly, which was being held together by staples and bandages.

In the room with my father, stepmother, and Lowell (my mother had gone home to rest), nurses and aides bustled about. June sat on the bed at my feet. She looked pale, vulnerable, and in profound distress. I felt sorry for her.

"How is Andrea?" I asked.

"She isn't well," Lowell replied. Fighting back tears, he approached my side and took my hand.

"What's wrong with her?"

"They don't know exactly. She's down the hall, on a respirator."

I looked in June's direction and asked, "What happened?"

"I don't know," she answered.

It didn't seem odd to me that June, who was in charge of Andrea's birth and had, over the years, been in charge of thousands of other births, did not know what had happened. I believed her. I had just passed thirty-two grueling hours sharing some of the most intimate moments of my life with her. In her presence, I had regressed to rudimentary behaviors as all propriety vanished. I had voided my bowels before her very eyes while straining to push Andrea out. We were in this together. Surely, some act of God must have taken place that no mortal could control.

My thoughts shifted within minutes from ones of disbelief—This can't be true, There must be some mistake—to ones of rationality—I must get the facts, I must see what I can do. The professionals surrounding me, hovering about my bed, almost blocking my family's access to me, responded to our inquiries obliquely. Even Dr. Kembel, who stopped by briefly, looking defeated and crushed, said he had no idea what had gone wrong. Everyone who was involved, during either the labor or the birth, appeared morose and somber, seemingly in shock at this thoroughly unexpected turn of events.

It was as if this roomful of people had encountered a phenomenon that was beyond their experience, and they had no reference points from which to extract reactions. We were all dumbfounded, humbled by the terror of the unknown. But I couldn't think about what had gone wrong; I could only think about Andrea. What did she look like? Was she in pain? Would she be all right?

A man walked warily into the room and introduced himself as Dr. Sherman, the neonatologist currently responsible for Andrea's care, her condition being beyond the expertise of a pediatrician. With obvious difficulty he reported the facts in the vernacular. He explained that she was suffering from perinatal asphyxia, a loss of oxygen at or shortly before the time of birth. He said one of her lungs was punctured from the force of the resuscitation. She had had seizures, so she was receiving phenobarbital. I couldn't understand a lot of what he said, since much of his vocabulary was from the language of neonatology. When I asked about her Apgar scores, the measure of newborn vitality, he said he believed the readings were one, then two, then three. On a scale of one to ten, with ten being what every baby should be blessed with, her Apgars were devastating. He ended with the recommendation that she be transferred to the NICU of another hospital because their own facility, which normally could have handled Andrea's special needs, was temporarily understaffed.

I thought, "Oh my God, they are going to take her away from me, just when she needs me the most." Then I realized that the recommended hospital was where Leona worked. Looking at Dr. Sherman I said, "We know a nurse in the NICU there. Anyway, there doesn't seem to be any choice but to transfer her."

I asked him the question that was burning inside: "Doctor, is she going to be . . . Can she survive the . . . Will she be normal? I mean, what about her brain? Can she come out of this?"

"Infants are amazingly resilient, and all you can do is have hope. There is hope here. I have seen babies in worse shape than Andrea come out okay." And he left to get the necessary papers for me to sign.

My anxieties were not relieved.

Soon after, a comparatively cheerful nurse appeared to wheel me down the hall to see Andrea. I had wanted to see her earlier, but for reasons that weren't clear to me, I couldn't. Lowell had been with her on and off, and he tried to prepare me.

"Honey, she's got these wires and things and something in her mouth. She's a little swollen in places, but she's beautiful. She's a little angel."

With Lowell beside me, I traveled down the corridor trying to restrain my excitement, dragging along the pole from which dangled my intravenous nutrition. So far I had managed to stay composed, detached, and numb; but then, I hadn't yet seen the child who was my daughter.

With much jolting of the wheelchair, which triggered excruciating pangs from my incision (the Demerol was wearing off), they managed to squeeze me into the tiny room used as an intensive care nursery.

Andrea lay on a cotton blanket on her back in an open container with clear plastic sides, her legs splayed open. She was at my eye level, and I had to stretch my upper torso to look down on her. She had thick black hair that was tousled above her closed eyes. Wide swaths of white masking tape encircled her lips, holding in place the mouthpiece and thick blue tube that connected her to the respirator. Little round suction cup–like things with wires adhered to several parts of her body, and the wires were attached to a monitor box with lights that blinked on and off. Protruding from her hand and from the ball of her foot were needles, also secured by masking tape, that looked gargantuan compared to her smallness. Her pinkish skin was stained brown by an antibacterial solution surrounding the masking tape that covered so much of her body. Her limbs and face were indeed swollen, and she had a vacant look, like a mangled doll with a mechanical apparatus that puffed out its chest.

Mute for the minutes it took to absorb the sight of her, I finally began to sob, with such force that waves of pain spread from my incision and I had to stop. I held back my tears, which could have poured out unceasingly. Physically, it hurt too much to cry.

Lowell, weeping himself, tried to comfort me, "Deb, she looks worse than she is. She's been through a trauma. She needs time to come around."

"Lowell, I hope to God you're right."

I wanted to touch her, but I didn't know if that was allowed. I felt intimidated by the machines, by the unnaturalness of her appearance. I was at a loss, and I did nothing.

My mother was in my room when I returned from the nursery. She came to me, hugging me in the wheelchair as best she could. Her fear of the worst and her hope for the best were written all over her face. She had seen Andrea, and she knew that she was to be transferred. She stood beside me stroking my head like she used to do when I was a child.

"Mom, this is so awful. I can't believe that that baby I just saw is Andrea. I'm afraid. I don't know how she can survive. I don't know how I'm going to survive. And Lowell, I feel so badly for him. Oh God, what is going to happen?"

Crying, she said over and over again, "I know, I know, I know."

Maintaining intimacy was awkward as nurses, aides, and midwives paraded through the room, checking my vital signs. Their activity kept my family and me from discussion. June urged, "You should start pumping your breast milk as soon as it comes so you don't get engorged."

"What should I do about that? I was planning on breast-feeding."

"You can always save the milk, freeze it if necessary, until the baby is ready for it," she replied.

I had just seen an infant who looked almost dead, and here we were talking about breast-feeding. How could this be? My whole orientation suddenly shifted, and I thought, "Are things not as bad as they seem? Is it possible that she'll be all right?" I knew that drugs taken by a nursing mother go right through her system and into her breast milk. I decided to take the absolute minimal amount of painkillers.

Yet another doctor whom I had never seen before entered my room to tell me that Andrea would be leaving soon by ambulance for the hospital across town.

"I'd like to see her before she goes."

They rolled her in, still in her isolette, still asleep. I had the head of my bed raised so I could get a good look at her. No matter how much I stared, I could not tell what she looked like, or whom she looked like. I told myself that I wouldn't break down, that I'd be strong. In my thoughts, as if I believed in telepathy, I told her that I loved her, that every-thing would be all right, and that I would recuperate as soon as possible so that I could come to her.

My exhausted parents all went home, and Lowell made a trip to our apartment to rest and get some things that we needed, including my journal. There was a daybed in the hospital room, which he would use that night. After every-one had gone I tried to sleep, but I was too troubled. Instead I simply lay there, drifting in and out of consciousness, gradually being consumed by a sadness so heavy that it felt like a presence with which I was merging.

That evening, while Lowell was away, I called the NICU. I learned that Andrea had had a seizure upon arriving at the hospital, for which she was given a massive dose of pheno-barbital. She was still on the respirator, though she had taken a few spontaneous breaths. Over the next few days she would have an EEG (electroencephalogram, to record electrical activity in the brain) and a CAT scan (an X-ray of her head to detect hemorrhages). There was nothing else they could tell me. I hung up the phone feeling utterly helpless.

Then someone I knew peeked his head into my room: Dr. Minsky, the pediatrician we had chosen for our daughter-to-be. I had last seen him at the end of my seventh month of pregnancy, when Lowell and I had consulted with him and his assistant, Evelyn, a nurse practitioner. We had been drawn to them both, agreeing without hesitation to have them care for our child. Dr. Minsky was a soft-spoken man who chose his words carefully and expressed himself slowly, always making sure that he was understood. He had children of his own, and he exuded a kindness so authentic that he seemed almost maternal, but without being feminine. Evelyn, a grandmother, was also warm, gentle, and experienced with infants and children. I had anticipated that it would be Dr. Minsky who would examine Andrea upon her birth.

As I beckoned him into the room he said, "Deborah, no one informed me of what was going on. I'm so sorry. Is there anything I can do?"

I told him that I had just called the hospital, and relayed the information I had been given. He already knew all this, though, having finally tracked Andrea down and spoken with the neonatologist in charge.

"Dr. Minsky, what are her chances? What do you think? What is your opinion, professionally, from what you know? Is it possible for her to have gone through this, to be having seizures . . . is it humanly possible for her to recover?"

"Deborah, it is humanly possible for her to pull out of this and be normal. Babies have had seizures and survived intact. The first forty-eight hours are crucial. She's getting excellent care, and she's where she should be. We can only wait and see."

It seemed hard for him to leave me. What could he say? What could anyone say?

I thought, "All I can do is pray and have faith." But to whom, and in what? I didn't believe in God.

I was awakened by a nurse who took my temperature and checked my pulse. I couldn't believe that she had disturbed me from the sleep I so desperately craved. I felt stiff, uncomfortable, disoriented. It was dark, and I could hear the muffled sounds of activity in the hallway. For a fleeting moment I didn't know where I was, but then the reality of what had happened seized my awareness, and I felt a chill penetrate my body. In the blackness, I saw Lowell asleep on the bed that wasn't long enough for his six-foot frame. I was grateful that he was there with me (I didn't remember his return from the apartment), though I knew he must be having a cramped and restless night. I watched him sleep and felt so sorry that his joyous expectancy had been destroyed. Now, not only did he have a daughter whose future was uncertain, but he also had me, currently incapacitated, to worry about.

As dawn gradually filtered through the closed blinds, sending cords of light throughout the room, I listened to the sounds of nurses ending and beginning their shifts and watched Lowell begin to stir. I was anxious to use the phone to call the NICU. I wondered if Andrea had made it through the night.

Before Lowell went out for breakfast, I made my call. "West-One," a voice answered.

"This is Deborah Alecson. I'm calling to find out how my daughter, Andrea, is doing." Using the term "daughter" seemed surreal. I was put on hold while the attending nurse came to the phone.

"Hello, Mrs. Alecson, this is Julie. I just got on. What would you like to know?"

"Well, how is she?" What I really wanted to know was if she had regained the perfection she had had when she was still a fetus. I wanted to hear that she was completely healed. What I heard instead were numbers referring to respirator settings, phenobarbital levels, and degrees of response to stimulation.

I asked, "Is she awake? Have her eyes opened? Is she looking around?" I wanted it to be me and not a stranger standing before her when she opened her eyes for the first time and saw the world into which she had been born.

"She's been sleeping. The phenobarbital level is still very

high. We have to wait till it reaches therapeutic level to see how she is. It's probably knocking her out.''

"What's therapeutic level?" I asked, wanting to know the magic moment when she'd wake up like a Sleeping Beauty who has been kissed.

"Between fifteen and thirty."

She gave me the names of Andrea's current doctors (they were always rotating), and we discussed when I could expect to speak with them. Then, feeling guilty, I explained, "I'm at the hospital recuperating from a C-section; otherwise I'd be there now. My husband will be coming by this morning." I concluded our conversation with the question I had asked everyone: "Does she seem to be in any kind of pain?"

"No," the nurse replied. This was what I was always told, but I never felt convinced.

During one of the rare moments when I was alone, after Lowell had left to see Andrea, I acknowledged a feeling I had, one I could only identify as shame. It was a subtle yet pervasive sense that I had done something wrong or had disgraced myself in some way. I felt as if I had failed, that I was a failure, that I had let Lowell and my family down. It was too disturbing to dwell on.

The big thrills of the morning were having the catheter removed, urinating twice on my own, and walking around the room. When the Demerol wore off I remained in distracting discomfort, but I was trying to go seven hours without having more. Thank goodness June persuaded me that four-hour intervals were long enough.

At one point she had come into my room visibly upset, fighting back tears, and I found myself comforting her. She lamented, "I just don't know what went wrong during that trip from the labor room to the operating room."

Lowell came back from seeing Andrea. He had met

Leona, who introduced him to the staff and helped him adjust to the place. She didn't have to be there, since she was still on leave, taking care of her baby. We hadn't known each other that long. Yet this was an emotionally wrenching situation. Her support was an act of kindness.

Lowell reported that Andrea was breathing on her own, and the seizures had abated. With this news of Andrea's independence, I let myself feel a guarded optimism. Maybe things weren't as bleak as they seemed. And Lowell didn't seem ravaged by his visit with her. Maybe all his running around between hospitals and our apartment was giving him a sense of purpose and control.

I wanted to hear all about Andrea and the NICU, but the hospital social worker was ready to talk with Lowell, my mother (who also was shuttling between hospitals), and me. This woman's cheerfulness struck me as fake and inappropriate. She passed the first minutes with us leafing through papers and organizing her pads. I could only surmise that she had a case load beyond anyone's capacity and, moreover, that she was simply unable, no matter how many graduate courses she had taken, to grasp the depth of our sorrow or the whys of our concern. I couldn't bear having to expose my grief to this woman who seemed so uncomfortable with the distress we emanated.

She said to me, "You look very upset," as if surprised.

I just looked at her, resenting the indignity of having to respond to such an inane observation.

Somehow we got through the interview, withholding our deepest regrets. Meanwhile, one emotion grew increasingly dominant: anger. I was angry that the privacy of my suffering would be converted into little comments in my hospital record. My mother was angry that the hospital hadn't provided us with a social worker to whom we felt we could relate. And Lowell, too, was angry, though I wasn't sure just why.

There was a knock at the door (which the social worker had closed). It was Sheila, a dear old friend and one of the few people I had called after the birth. While my mother and I tried to end the meeting with the social worker, Lowell led Sheila to the lounge, where he described what had been going on since I had spoken to her.

She was shaky when she returned, carefully embracing me and giving me a bouquet of lilacs. She said, "I didn't know what to bring."

"I love lilacs," I assured her. "They're my favorite flower."

Sheila had a history of mental breakdowns, and I knew that she was struggling with this crisis she had walked into, a situation that could rattle her in ways neither of us could predict. But I couldn't protect her by modifying the circumstances or by pretending not to be distressed.

I showed her the photo I had of Andrea, barely visible beneath the tubes and wires, a Polaroid taken by one of the nurses before she was transferred. "Here's my baby," I said, hearing the anger in my voice.

The phone rang. It was my father to tell me that he had gotten in touch with a bigwig at the new hospital and that this doctor would be looking out for Andrea. My father had many connections with people who ran corporations, hospitals, the government, and a myriad social and philanthropic institutions from when he was a bigwig himself at one of the largest nonprofit organizations in the country. Though he had retired from that world, he maintained some ties with people of influence. It seemed to me, though, that only the bigwig in the sky could help Andrea now. Still, I certainly valued my father's networking. It was his way of trying to help, of trying to do something.

When I told him that June had come to visit and that she was despondent and always near tears, he became angry.

"Deb, that woman is dumping on you. You don't need her coming around being sad and miserable."

"Dad, I don't think you're being fair. She's almost as upset as I am."

"I want to tell you something, Deb. Kitty and I don't trust her or Dr. Kembel. We think they know much more than they're letting on. Has Lowell talked to you about any of this?"

"No."

"Well, Lowell has talked to us. I think you should be very careful around her."

The thought that June could be concealing something from us was so incompatible with my loyalty to her that I couldn't assimilate what my father was saying. I told him that I had a visitor and we'd talk later.

Shuffling across the room, I told Sheila about the labor and what I knew about the birth. She seemed distracted and pained, as if my very words were tormenting her. She interrupted to tell me she had to go. "I don't know what to say. What to do," she said. "It's too much for me. I hope you understand." And she fled the room.

I did understand.

That night before going to sleep, I remembered that I hadn't told Lowell about the phone conversation with my father. During the few private moments we did have, we talked about Andrea and the treatment she was receiving at the NICU. My father's suspicions were unsettling, though. I pushed them aside and replaced them with words I had heard Dr. Minsky use earlier that day. He had said that "hope is grounded" because the sonogram of Andrea's head was normal and she was still breathing on her own. At this stage, however, a normal sonogram was to be expected.

Lowell went to see Andrea first thing in the morning, leaving me to attend to my appearance. I felt like a mess.

With the intravenous still intact, pole in tow, I managed to shower and wash my hair. I put on a fresh hospital gown and prepared myself for my first walk outside the room. I had before me the intestinal goals of, first, passing gas, and then having a bowel movement. These two bodily functions would lead to my being disconnected from the intravenous and getting real food—all of which ultimately meant being released from the hospital.

I had been hearing the lusty cries of newborns throughout my stay, but now I saw the babies belonging to those cries. Although I avoided the nursery, I couldn't help but pass the rooms of new mothers with their infants in their arms, surrounded by oohing and aahing relatives. It was unbearable to witness; yet I found myself pausing more than once before an open door, watching intently the intimate and tender interactions I was not privy to. It made me more determined than ever to get out of the hospital and be with Andrea.

When I returned from my trip I found Lucy in my room setting up the breast pump. It was my first encounter with this intimidating apparatus, which could have been some kind of vacuum cleaner, for all I knew. Lucy helped me get comfortable in a chair and showed me how to fit the cone-shaped funnel onto my nipple and adjust the strength of suction. The pump itself was soothingly rhythmic, and the tugging on my breast was not unpleasant. To my amazement, liquid began to squirt out and then flow. It was coming out of me! It was my milk! It felt like a miracle was taking place. Lucy had told me that the more milk you express, the more milk you will continue to produce. At that point, though, all I wanted was to relieve the pressure.

I was sitting in bed after my second tour of the floor when Lowell returned from seeing Andrea.

''Deb, she's back on the respirator.''

I started to cry, a steady and silent stream of tears as I clutched the sides of the bed to keep still.

"Honey, they said this kind of thing happens. She may be back off it tonight. It's two steps forward, one step back."

I had to stop my tears dead in their tracks; I simply could not bear a quivering belly. The Demerol had been replaced by Tylenol with codeine, a not very effective substitute.

To keep me from obsessing over this setback, he talked about the NICU and about one of the nurses he especially liked, Gloria. She had washed Andrea's hair and attached a little white bow to one of the probes that was fastened to her skull. The touches she added to Andrea's person reminded Lowell of her babyhood, her sweetness, her innocence. Lowell spoke of the NICU and of Andrea's condition with increasing familiarity, and I was a little jealous of his presence in Andrea's life. He was already acting in the capacity of a father, despite all the barriers, while I was stuck in the hospital, miles away from my daughter, waiting to have a goddamn bowel movement.

The afternoon passed with phone calls from relatives as the news of our calamity spread throughout our families. My mother's sister and her husband wanted to visit me and bring my grandparents. I didn't know if I was ready to face them, to play host from my hospital bed. I felt pretty unstable, and I didn't want to burden my grandparents with a despair I couldn't conceal. Nevertheless, I told my aunt that if they were all willing to make the trip from Brooklyn, I'd certainly welcome them. I knew that my grandparents were worried about me and that they needed to see that I was all right and in one piece.

My father called from his place upstate. He asked, "Are you depressed?" as if I had no reason to be. Obviously, he wanted me to sound upbeat, even if I didn't feel that way. I was angry with him when we hung up. In effect, he had lectured me on how I should feel—that is, in a way that would make him feel comfortable and safe from his own grief. My mother, meanwhile, was visiting Andrea, touching her, looking for signs of response. When we last had spoken I said, "I want to hold my baby." She just cried and kept repeating, "Oh my God, oh my God."

A big surprise arrived: a bouquet of flowers from Lowell's parents and his sister's family with a card that read, "Congratulations!" If they had come from anyone else, I would have judged these tokens as cruel and insensitive. Lowell had spoken to his parents, who lived in Minnesota, and he said they felt badly and hoped that everything would be all right. Being separated by a distance of twelve hundred miles and not knowing how else to respond, they did "the right thing" and sent flowers. To me, those gorgeously fragrant blossoms were a reminder of a happy occasion gone wrong; but Lowell's family could never understand that. I couldn't be upset with them; indeed, there was something so typical and predictable about their gesture that I could almost appreciate its absurdity.

I also spoke with Sheila, who explained her abrupt departure. "I was just so overwhelmed with emotion," she said.

That afternoon, too, I was sitting on the edge of my bed when I looked up to find Dr. Minsky in the doorway. I told him that Andrea was back on the respirator, which he knew, and then I started to cry—really cry. He sat beside me on the bed while I clutched my belly and tried to keep it from shaking. He rubbed my back, enabling me to let go even more. When I finally stopped, aware that that was the first "good" cry I'd had since Andrea's birth, I felt indebted to him.

My family never made it that evening. My aunt called, terribly disturbed, unable to find the right words, and said that they'd come tomorrow. I talked Lowell out of going to pay Andrea a second visit. He was exhausted, and we needed time together.

Gently, and with great caution, we managed to lie side by side on my bed. We clung to each other, discussing our concerns. We agreed to keep on having hope while not denying the horrendous possibilities. We even talked about life after my discharge from the hospital. Lowell wanted to give voice lessons to a few choice students. I wasn't so sure about that.

"On the one hand, it would be good for you to get back to as normal a life as possible. On the other, it isn't good for us to have to put up a front."

One of our friends had said, "If there is anything I can do for you . . ." What he could do, Lowell said, was let Lowell teach at his apartment, thus sparing me the intrusions.

"Lowell, it's so strange to be talking about the things we were involved with before Andrea. I can't imagine how our lives are going to continue as they have. Can you?"

"No. Everything's different now. I can't believe that I'll have to go back to work."

We held each other and cried. Before going to sleep I called the NICU for the evening report. A nurse named Cheryl said Andrea's phenobarbital level was at forty-nine, and she moved her foot when touched. "She's a little more responsive," she said, which made me ask, "Does she seem uncomfortable in any way?"

"She's asleep, Mrs. Alecson, and very calm."

Calm—that's a nice way of describing comatose. I always felt disappointed after my calls to the NICU because I was never told what I wanted to hear.

Lowell and I imagined, for a moment, trying to sleep together on my bed but quickly abandoned the idea. Not only was it a single, but I was still in great discomfort.

I had a violent start in the morning when I got up to go

to the bathroom. I was suddenly overcome by chills. I called out to Lowell, asleep on the daybed, to get a nurse. After taking my temperature, which was normal, the nurse covered me with a heated blanket and piled on more blankets; but it took a long time before I warmed up. The shivering was apparently a result of my moving too quickly and of the let-down of my breast milk. There must have been a connection between that shock to my system and the events I was waiting for, because soon I finally passed gas and had some diarrhea. I immediately asked for the lunch menu. After perusing the dismal selection, I asked Lowell to get me a massive muffin from my favorite deli.

It was quiet on the ward, which seemed empty of staff. Before going to see Andrea, Lowell helped me deal with an engorged right breast, which was sending searing pains throughout my body. He improvised compresses, running washcloths under hot tap water.

Lowell got back from the NICU just as Dr. Kembel arrived to remove my staples. The sight of Dr. Kembel triggered panic, then dread. I felt a repulsion that I couldn't explain, which made his treatment of my incision an odious thing to endure. Managing to keep my feelings to myself, I asked, ''Dr. Kembel, when is the absolute earliest I can be discharged?''

Methodically snipping, as if my belly was zippered shut, he answered, ''Normally, Tuesday, but under the circumstances, since I know how much you want to see your baby, you can leave tomorrow.''

''Thank you. That was all I wanted to hear.''

Then he asked about Andrea, as he always did after checking in on me.

Lowell walked out of my room with the doctor, and I burst into tears. I explained my reaction to Kembel as the association I made between him and the turn for the worse of my labor.

When Lowell returned, though, he announced, "Deb, I'm getting all your records and Andrea's before you leave this hospital. I haven't spoken to you about this, but I've spoken to your father, and I feel very angry at Kembel. Your father agrees with me, but we haven't wanted to get you involved because we don't want you to get more upset. I'll handle this for now."

I told him about my visceral reaction upon seeing Kembel and how frightening it was.

The distrust I felt for my doctor aroused a powerful emotional dichotomy, for I still needed him to attend to my body. It was almost like being a child who, for reasons of survival, cannot reject abusive parents.

That evening we were treated to the hospital's special dinner of filet mignon and a rich dessert, given to all maternity patients and their spouses the night before discharge. It was supposed to be a celebratory meal, but I hadn't the stomach for it.

My aunt, uncle, and grandparents finally came. Uncle Howie slipped me forty dollars for the cab ride to see Andrea (I planned to go straight from my hospital bed to hers). Grandma alternated between complete denial of the circumstances as she commented incessantly about the room, and a silent sadness. Aunt Selma was the only one who asked about and listened to all that had transpired. She said, shaking her head, "Get everything in writing. None of this sounds right."

First thing the next morning, I spoke to Gloria. "She's stable, breathing a little on her own. The phenobarbital level is at fifty-one, and she responds to stimulation. I'm getting her ready for your visit."

I had woken up feeling strong and purposeful. I called Sheila to see if she'd come by to help us get my things home. She said she would; I knew she wouldn't let us down.

June, at my request, spoke to us for a while, and I was

satisfied with her report and recollections, though they did not explain how my uneventful labor had turned so suddenly into a crisis. Lowell, on his own, asked that June show him copies of the charts and records before I was discharged. He also spoke with Dr. Kembel. He felt concerned about apparent differences between Kembel's evaluation and June's. Just when, exactly, Andrea had become endangered, and whether the Caesarean was at first perceived to be an emergency, remained unclear.

As I packed, Lowell went to the administrative offices. He was tense and raging inside. Although he had always been uncomfortable realizing, accepting, and expressing his anger, now he was clearly in touch with it and directing it toward the people he believed deserved it: Dr. Kembel and June.

While waiting for Lowell and Sheila to return from our apartment to then lead me out the door of the hospital, I sat on the bed, nervous in anticipation of seeing Andrea, and wrote in my journal: "Will it turn out that it would have been better if she had died?"

3

Hope

The taxi ride was a miserable journey of jolts, sudden stops, and endless potholes. I thought my incision would split open.

At the hospital, Lowell led the way through lobbies, corridors, banks of elevators, and hallways to reach West-One. Before entering the nursery, we had to scrub our hands and don yellow disposable gowns over our clothes. Once aseptic, we activated the sliding glass doors and entered what could very well have been a spaceship.

Although Lowell had described the NICU, I wasn't prepared for that electric universe of tiny creatures, some barely recognizable as human, who lay in transparent vessels dormant, or in varying degrees of contortion. Many looked like the fetuses I had seen in photographs, but instead of floating in amniotic fluid, curled and buffered against external stimuli, they were removed from the womb and exposed to the world. It wasn't a world of human scent, mother's flesh, and familiar voices. It was a world of perpetual light and an incessant drone of uterine machines that periodically signaled danger or distress with a high-pitched ringing. Attending to those minuscule patients were busy giants who adjusted parts of machinery taped onto, stuck into, and wrapped around their translucent bodies, while regulating their flow of aliments, wastes, and secretions with tubes and suctioning devices.

When I first saw Andrea, with Lowell and Gloria (her primary nurse) at my side, I felt my blood drain. There was all the apparatus I had seen before, plus additional probes fixed to her scalp, which was shaved to allow for adhesion. Her belly button was black with dried blood: the crumbling of her umbilical stump. A catheter was inserted into her puffy vagina. She was totally enmeshed in a tangle of wires and plastic tubes that extended outside the isolette. The criticalness of her condition so assaulted me that if Gloria hadn't brought me a chair, I would have collapsed.

I sat, speechless, looking at Andrea and sensed a paralysis creep through my body. Lowell leaned over the isolette and began talking to her: "Hello, Andrea, this is Daddy. Your momma's here too." I watched Lowell being a father, reaching out to our baby, while I sat, self-conscious and inept.

But that sense of impotence passed, and was replaced with a longing to make contact with her. I stood up, shaky in the knees, stuck my arms through the portholes as Lowell had, and was astonished when her fingers closed around my thumb.

"Would you mind if I had a few moments alone with her?" I asked, needing to get my bearings.

"Of course not. I'll wait over there." He pointed to a lounge on the other side of the nursery.

Overcoming my shyness, I finally was able to speak.

"Andrea, this is Mommy. I don't even know if you can hear me or are aware of my presence but I want you to know that I love you. And I'm sorry this has happened. Oh God, I'm so sorry this has happened.''

I hadn't wanted to cry because I was afraid that once I started, I'd never stop. But the tears came, and, blocking out everything around us, I concentrated on Andrea, scrutinizing every aspect of her. Behind the adhesive tape and sensors and collection of cords was my beautiful daughter, who looked healthy and plump. She had a pug nose that neither Lowell nor I possessed, but her forehead was shaped in the classic Alecson mode: high and wide. I thought, ''She would have been flawless from her sweet face to her perfect little toes. To think that once my greatest concern was that she should start life out on my chest, sucking. That certainly turned out to be the least of it.''

Lowell returned with Gloria, who, in the gentlest voice, asked if I'd like to hold Andrea.

''Of course I would, but I can't yet. I'm really in agony from the Caesarean, and I couldn't manage her in my lap. Maybe tomorrow.''

Within minutes of meeting Gloria, I trusted her. Her cherubic face was open, her gray eyes kind, and her demeanor self-assured. She showed Lowell and me the same compassion she showed Andrea. In her arms, I imagined the healing of countless babies and the comforting of their weeping mothers and fathers. In that environment of technological wizardry, I was relieved to know that such a loving human being would be, in effect, taking my place as Andrea's caregiver.

We talked about Leona, how I knew her, and under what circumstances we had met. I didn't mention to Gloria that I believed that my acquaintanceship with Leona would help us get what we needed for Andrea. Not that Andrea would be given priority over the other babies, but that Lowell and I would be treated by the staff as more real, so to speak, than if we were complete strangers, "just another couple" with an impaired newborn on West-One. Our situation was closer to home for this tightly knit unit because we had a relationship with one of their own.

"Gloria, is there anything else you can tell us about Andrea?" I asked.

"I wish I could, but there's nothing anyone can tell you until after the tests. And they can't be done until the phenobarbital level goes down. I know it's hard, but you'll have to wait and be patient."

Being patient while waiting was an ability that I did not have. Patience only compounded the lack of power I felt from having to wait. I had waited to get pregnant. I had waited nine months for Andrea to be born. And now I had to wait for some drug in her system to dissipate. Then I'd have to wait for tests to be performed, and wait again for the results.

The day was taking its toll, and I felt depleted. In addition, my breasts were becoming increasingly full and achy. When I mentioned this to Gloria, she told me I could pump them there. She led me to a makeshift tentlike compartment that housed one chair, an electric pump, and a couple of cardboard cartons filled with plastic funnels, bottles, and tubes and glass jars of sterilized water. The public telephone was adjacent to this cubbyhole, and the "family lounge" was right outside. With one vigorous jerk of an arm from within, I soon learned, the cloth "door" could open, thus displaying a lactating mother, naked from the waist up, the wheezing machine sucking out her milk. Gloria left me within this chamber to do my thing, and I fumbled my way through it, conscious always of the men and women on the other side of the curtain who heard, I was certain, every squirt. After seven minutes pumping each breast, I poured the precious extract into specially designed freezer bags, which I proudly handed to Gloria to store.

I took one last look at Andrea before leaving for the day. I told myself that all I could do was have faith that she was where she belonged and that our separation was not harming her further.

"Goodbye, sweet baby. I'll see you tomorrow."

At home, our answering machine blinked with messages from friends and family. We hadn't the stamina to share our heartbreak with those who were calling about a bundle of joy. I had my things to unpack, and I had to rest. There was a message from June, returning Lowell's call. He was still trying to get the hospital records and fetal monitor strips. She inquired after our well-being and suggested a time when she could meet with Lowell.

I did call Rhonda back, with whom Lowell and I had been in contact since Andrea's birth.

"Deb, I can arrange to be free tomorrow. What is it you need me to do? I'm putting myself at your disposal."

We decided that she should come to our apartment in the morning and accompany me to the NICU.

"I have to warn you, you will be shocked when you see Andrea."

"Deborah, please, don't worry about me. I can handle it. I love you. I'll see you tomorrow."

Lowell and I rummaged through the refrigerator for enough food to make a meal, but neither of us could eat. We moved about our apartment like somnambulists, opening mail then leaving it unread, incapable of even putting a grocery list together. I avoided the nursery, in which stood the cradle we had borrowed, all prepared for Andrea with a pink sheet and a teddy bear.

Before going to bed, my breasts had to be pumped. I had

purchased a simple hand pump at our local pharmacy. It had two plastic cylinders: one slid into the other, with a cone at the end to be placed over the nipple. It required the kind of pumping action used to inflate bicycle tires. I sat on the edge of the couch and began to get a momentum going, but the milk wasn't expressing with the effusion I had experienced with the hospital's pump. I was working up a sweat, and my arms were getting tired. I became hysterical and wrenched the contraption from my chest, hurling it across the living room.

"This fucking thing doesn't work. On top of everything else, I'm going to have engorged breasts that will turn to rocks overnight," I cried out. Retrieving the gadget from behind a chair, I tried to crack the cylinders in two with my hands as droplets of milk leaked from my breasts onto my lap.

Lowell sat beside me on the couch and calmed me down. Then, with steady concentration, I managed to relieve the lactation buildup enough to ensure some hours of comfort through the night.

In bed, in each other's arms, we told ourselves that there was a chance she'd be all right and that we'd hope for that. But if it turned out that she wouldn't be all right and that her existence would be a living hell for her and for us, we would not wish that heroic measures be taken to prolong her life. We were of one heart and mind; we agreed that the quality of Andrea's life had to be considered. Then we slipped into exhausted, restless sleep.

The next morning on our way to the hospital, Rhonda shared an incredible family story in response to my doubts that Andrea would emerge unscathed. She told me about her aunt, whose second child was born with massive damage to the nervous system. "My aunt left the hospital and deserted the baby. Her husband's brother, who had money, made arrangements for the baby. The whole thing was never discussed.''

"Did she have more kids?" I asked.

"Yes, as a matter of fact, she did have one more. The child was fine.''

"Rhonda, I can't believe she could do that, that she could just walk out and never find out what became of her child.''

"Look, I'm not saying it was right or wrong. I don't know. It did take a certain courage. After all, she couldn't do anything for the baby, who, from what I understand, would have been a vegetable. She said she had to do it to preserve the family.''

"If it came to the point that I would have to consider abandoning Andrea, I don't know what I'd do. It's more than I can bear to think about.''

As difficult as this discussion was for me, it was also a relief. To find language for the inexpressible gives it a certain reality. Abandoning one's baby under extraordinary cir-cumstances could be seen as altruistic. Things are not all black and white. I had always felt that Rhonda viewed the world from a larger perspective than most people I knew, and her morality was based on thoughtful conclusions she reached about an examined life. I could articulate the un-thinkable, and she'd accept it for what it was: a projection into the unknown.

We arrived at the NICU to find Andrea lying on a diaper without the catheter. The sight of the diaper brought tears of joy to my eyes. Diapers are what normal babies have.

"Deborah, she's beautiful. Like a little doll,'' Rhonda exclaimed, her eyes brimming with tears.

There was a thin tube extending out of one of her nostrils. When Gloria joined us, I asked about it.

"That's a nasogastric tube and it runs directly into her

stomach. You'll be pleased to know that we gave her some of your breast milk, which she tolerated fairly well.''

I thought, "My breast milk. Wow. She's getting what she needs from me after all." Then I asked, "Doesn't that thing bother her? Isn't it uncomfortable?"

"We don't think so. Besides, it is most important now that she receive nutrition in any way possible."

Rhonda was absorbing every detail of the place and of Andrea's neighbors, who were the smallest babies she had ever seen. "Deb, I feel like we've entered a foreign world. This is a separate reality from my conscious life, that's for sure."

I had my hand through a porthole and was stroking Andrea's body. Rhonda reached in too and touched her hand. It responded with a flutter. Rhonda, who was aware of a sacred dimension to life, said she felt the emanation of Andrea's soul. She sensed her spirit.

We were interrupted by the nurse practitioner, Gloria, who said the attending neonatologist, Dr. Hines, was available to speak with me. I asked Rhonda to be present, for I expected some kind of news.

We walked into a cubicle of an office shared by two doctors, who were separated by a simple divider. Since I could hear every word of the other doctor's conversation on the phone, I was sure she would be able to hear every word of ours. I told Dr. Hines, a slight blond man with blue eyes and a tan, that I'd like some privacy, if possible. He in turn was hesitant about having Rhonda present, since she wasn't immediate family. Nevertheless, he accommodated me by allowing her to stay, and he assured me that his office mate was about to leave.

Dr. Hines remained silent for a long time, which made me uncomfortable and confused, as if I was the one who had asked to meet and so should speak first. When he finally did speak, what he said was vague and noncommital, his few words delivered with an unreadable facial expression.

"We have to wait until the phenobarbital wears off before we can give her a CAT and an EEG. Then we'll know something."

"You must have some ideas," I said. "I mean, you must have had babies in her condition before. Can you tell me if it is at all possible that she can recover?"

"We can't determine anything just yet."

"You're telling me that you haven't anything to say whatsoever?"

"Yes."

Rhonda, recognizing an impatience on my part that was expanding into exasperation, intervened. "Deb, he would tell you something if he could. You don't want him to make guesses. Meet again after the tests."

When would the phenobarbital go down enough to do the tests? This he couldn't tell me either.

I left the meeting feeling vexed and incredulous that nothing could be determined by a physical examination and by careful observation. What value did Dr. Hines derive from a meeting in which he couldn't or wouldn't reveal what he thought or felt?

When we returned to Andrea's isolette, Gloria was tidying her up.

"Can I hold her now?" I asked.

"Absolutely, but let's first get a chair for you."

Nervously, I watched Gloria open the isolette and lift Andrea out. There were so many contraptions to keep from becoming unattached or intertwined, and, much to my horror, she disconnected the respirator tube for the few seconds it took to place Andrea on my lap. My incision was still a source of great pain, so it took some shifting around before I was comfortable.

The world around me vanished as I focused on Andrea. She was real! She was alive! I touched every part of her and talked in a hush, "Hello my sweet baby. This is Momma. I'm holding you now. I've been wanting to hold you for so long." I began to sob. Her eyes were sealed shut and she did not make a sound, though she did tighten her fingers around one of mine. I fell into a trance; time became suspended. Then my father and stepmother appeared and quietly approached. Kitty put her arm around my shoulders; my father stood to the side. They studied her while I stroked her face. We did not speak.

Gloria returned to tell me my time was up and that Andrea had to go back in. Kissing her forehead, I said goodbye.

I needed to cry some more, but I didn't want to do it in front of my father. He had always been uncomfortable with emotionalism, and I didn't want to have to consider his sensitivities at this time. I excused myself to use the hospital pump, leaving Rhonda, my father, and Kitty outside the nursery to talk.

My father drove me home in his van, but first I wanted to go to the one pharmacy I knew of that rented breast pumps. It was rush hour, the pharmacy was about to close, and my physical misery was heightened because of the active day. What little progress we did make along the streets of Manhattan came to a halt when we encountered a garbage truck obstructing traffic. As the truck sat idle, the two young workers scurried up and down the street collecting litter, thus adding thirty minutes to their cleanup of one block. My father, never one to tolerate inconvenience, began to rave about the ineptitude with which these fellows performed their jobs. This led to a discourse on the decay of New York

City, the incompetence of the people who ran it, and the inevitable deterioration of a once-proud city. Like many of his tirades, it was funny and sarcastic, and he kept me from mental collapse as I visualized our getting to the pharmacy after closing time. It was also easier for him to talk about his powerlessness before a city run amok than his powerlessness before his six-day-old granddaughter. He got out of the van and confronted the boys. I saw him gesticulating, pointing to the line of honking vehicles behind us. By the time he was back in the driver's seat the workers had moved the truck out of the way, and we proceeded.

We got to the pharmacy in the nick of time, and I rented the last pump available. I hadn't realized in what demand they were. There must have been women all over the city seated before breast pumps, bottling their milk.

My parents dropped me and the pump off at my apartment. Lowell was home, having given a voice lesson while I was at the hospital. He was managing to return to an aspect of his former life, before Andrea, and behave in a professional manner. He had shared with the student enough of our ordeal to keep him informed, but not so much as to upset him so that he couldn't open his mouth to sing. I knew that giving lessons again was healthy for Lowell, and I envied his ability to carry on. It was a small step into an arena that did not have Andrea at its center. He would be returning in a couple of days to the high school, where his students and fellow teachers would clamor for more news about our baby. With the private students, he could get practice telling Andrea's story without going to pieces.

We collapsed on the couch and played back our phone messages. One was from a Nancy Cronin, a lawyer and the daughter of a friend of my father's who just happened to be an obstetrician affiliated with Andrea's hospital. My father had spoken to this friend, Dr. Klein, about Andrea's birth and had asked if he had any influence at the hospital. He also wondered if there might be some negligence involved: that's when Nancy's name was brought up. Lowell and I had discussed the wisdom of talking with a lawyer and had decided that we should. I called Nancy and gave her an abbreviated account of the labor and birth. To my surprise, she responded with genuine empathy and concern. Perhaps because I had had no prior dealings with lawyers, I harbored a stereotypic picture of them; certainly, one of the qualities I did not associate with them was sensitivity. Nancy was willing to come to our place for a meeting, which further impressed me.

I also spoke with my former therapist, whom I hadn't seen as a patient in a number of years. We were, at this stage, friends. Since the day I'd met Dr. Melner, he was the one I called when I was in trouble. I had already spoken with him from my hospital bed, so he knew what was happening. I needed to have a session with him. I wanted to lose control, weep and wail, and dredge up all the feelings I was keeping suppressed. I had to do this with someone I trusted, with someone who could make sure I wouldn't go off the deep end. We made an appointment for the next week.

Once again it was time to eat dinner, and once again it was a trial. Chinese food was out of the question. Lowell now had an aversion to it after that chicken-with-broccoli meal he'd had while I sat laboring in the bathtub. Neither of us could get it together enough to prepare a meal. We were helpless. The old habits of familial life were disintegrating. We ordered a pizza and then just picked at it. Afterward, Lowell went to pay Andrea a nocturnal visit.

Before going to bed I sat at the pump, which we had set up in the nursery for want of a better location, and looked around the room we had created for our baby. I scanned the shelves filled with toys, stuffed animals, and books. A square flowered box of tissues sat unopened on her dresser. I could smell a faint baby odor emanating from the clothes Rhonda had given us, now stuffed in dresser drawers. I had bought lotion, cornstarch, Baby Wipes, and cotton swabs, which were in view. I took in the little home we had created for our beloved child, pumped my breasts, and cried.

At six the next morning, while I still slept, Lowell phoned the home number of the neonatologist who had been summoned upon Andrea's birth. It was audacious to call Dr. Sherman at such an ungodly hour, but the strain of our crisis was enabling both of us to act in ways that reticence, quiescence, and perhaps common sense had once constrained. Lowell had lain awake since four thinking about the chain of events that led up to Andrea's birth. He wanted to speak with the doctor who resuscitated her, and the only way he could think of to get the man's name and phone number was by calling Dr. Sherman.

When I woke up, Lowell told me about the phone call.

"My God, Lowell, you must have shocked the guy."

"He was half asleep, but when I introduced myself he became alert. I apologized for waking him."

"So, what did he say?"

"He gave me the doctor's name, Dr. Pedro, and said he'd call back later this morning when he's at his office."

"Lowell, that took chutzpah. I'm proud of you. He must think you're suspicious of something. I wonder if he plans to call Kembel and June?"

"I don't know. Deb, when I was at the hospital last night, Andrea couldn't tolerate the milk. So the feedings have stopped and the catheter is back in."

I burst into tears.

"Honey, we have to expect these setbacks. This is just the

beginning. Please . . .'' He held me in his arms until I was calm.

Lowell wanted to visit Andrea in the morning because he planned to meet with my father and Kitty in the afternoon. I needed to take a shower before he left, an undertaking that required Lowell's assistance. Preparing for it involved my nudity, Lowell's skills, and mutual cooperation, making it an almost erotic experience. His main task was to cut a rectangular piece of plastic from a dry-cleaning bag or a roll of Saran Wrap and tape it securely onto my abdomen to keep the incision from getting wet. Every time I wanted to shower, it would take at least fifteen minutes for him to fashion a neat parallelogram, place it just so, and seal it to my skin. Eighty percent of the time it would leak anyway, and I'd end up with a soggy plastic bag and sticky masking tape hanging from my body.

While I was waiting for Dr. Sherman's call, the diaper service arrived with a hefty stack of fifty cloth diapers, plus plastic bags and a rubber container in which to deposit used ones. I had forgotten about the order I'd put in a week before Andrea's due date. I explained to the delivery man that I wouldn't be needing the diapers. He said, ''Mrs. Alecson, it's my job to deliver them, so here they are. You can call the office to make a change.'' He had me sign a receipt, then he disappeared down the four flights of stairs.

I called and spoke with a woman who expressed sorrow for my situation but was unwilling to accept an unhappy ending. ''Hold on to them for a while. Your daughter will be home in no time,'' she urged. She didn't understand that the presence of those diapers was distressing for me.

''Believe me, my daughter will be in the hospital for a long time, and I would really prefer that my order be canceled and that someone pick these up.''

Reluctantly, she agreed to do as I asked. When I got off

the phone, I sat on the couch and stared at the diapers. I thought that her reaction was not about keeping a customer; rather, it was an inability to accept that unforeseen horrors do occur for which there are no explanations.

I dreaded having to tell people about what had happened and what was still happening to Andrea. Everyone in the neighborhood, in my building, and at the pool had seen me swell with pregnancy over the months, and now I was obviously fetus-free. At first, I evaded many chance encounters by crossing to the other side of the street. I avoided stores I had frequented and stayed away from the health club entirely. I did not want to upset people with the news that the baby we all assumed would be normal and healthy was in fact a disaster. Things weren't supposed to go wrong in this way. Childbirth was not supposed to be a life-threatening event for either mother or child anymore. I was an unsettling reminder that misfortune could strike at any time. Even more difficult than telling my story was contending with people's reactions, which could range from denial—"Surely she'll be perfectly fine"—to sympathy—"I'm so sorry"—to attempts to empathize—"I had a cousin who had a premature baby and . . ."

I felt fragile and unsure of myself. I didn't know how the retelling of my labor and the delivery would affect me.

When Dr. Sherman called, I grabbed a pad and pen. "Thank you for calling. You must have been surprised to hear from my husband. We've been pretty upset. The thing that is really unclear to us is if my Caesarean was an emergency and, if so, when it became one. Dr. Kembel says it was never an emergency. But in that case, why did I get general anesthesia and an incision that is far from cosmetic? June also says it wasn't an emergency. But then why wasn't Lowell in the operating room with me as June had promised? She tells us that Andrea had a normal heartbeat throughout. If that's true, why did she lose the heartbeat in the operating room?''

''The baby had a heartbeat of twelve to fourteen beats per minute,'' Dr. Sherman interrupted.

''What does that mean?''

''It's very bad. And she convulsed a half hour later.''

''Which means?''

''That the insult probably occurred hours earlier.''

''You're saying things went wrong while she was in the womb, while I was in labor?''

''That's what it looks like.''

''So it *was* an emergency. What can we do?''

''Let's meet tomorrow, and you and your husband can talk with Dr. Pedro, the pediatrician who resuscitated your daughter. Let's try to piece this all together.'' And we arranged for a late-morning meeting.

This conversation changed my way of thinking about everything and everyone. Instead of wondering to the heavens above how such a cruel fate could have befallen my baby, I began to examine the events leading up to the Caesarean section. For the first time I considered the possibility that someone's negligence had caused her damage, that it wasn't some freak accident or the result of something I'd done wrong.

My mother was beside Andrea's isolette when I came into the NICU. She had left work early to be with her. ''I needed to see her,'' she explained.

I so admired my mother for allowing herself to experience her granddaughter while knowing, as Lowell and I knew, that her future was uncertain. She didn't run away, and she didn't put herself on hold. She could understand my anguish because she had the courage to get in touch with her own.

I stood next to her and told her about my conversation with Dr. Sherman.

''Ma, I'm beginning to think there was a major fuck-up.''

''What does Lowell think?'' she asked while rubbing Andrea's toes through the porthole.

''Well, he's meeting later with Dad and Kitty to talk about everything. And we're also going to meet at our place with a lawyer, the daughter of a friend of Dad's who's an obstetrician at this hospital. I talked to this gal over the phone, and she wants to investigate further, to see if there may be some liability. I don't know. It's a whole other level. And what difference does it make anyway? Here's Andrea.''

''That's right. Here's Andrea.''

In silence we beheld this newborn lying in the deepest sleep, whose limbs would occasionally shudder, and her face, quiver. She was pure innocence, a celestial being suspended in a tiny body like light captured in a crystal.

At home there awaited a vegetarian casserole cooked by a former voice student of Lowell's who lived on our block. Lowell had run into her earlier in the day and told her about Andrea. Doreen wasn't a close friend, but she knew we had been expecting, and her apparent understanding of our grief and incapacitations was that of a sister or cousin. She took it upon herself to feed us, and not junk food thrown together in haste or made of leftovers from meals past, but a casserole that had taken skill and time to prepare, composed of organic, chemical-free ingredients. It was a generous offering that was totally unexpected and greatly appreciated—after all, we were hardly doing well in the meal department.

The downstairs buzzer rang; it was Nancy Cronin, right on time. I was momentarily conscious of the disarray our apartment was in and the untidiness of my own person. Lately I didn't think too clearly when I dressed in the mornings, and I didn't have many clothes that fit my post-pregnant self anyway. ''It's too late to straighten up,'' I thought as I opened the front door.

There stood Nancy, dressed in full Wall Street regalia: a beige tailored suit, white silk blouse, beige pumps, attaché case, and the largest diamond I had ever seen, glittering in its setting. She looked much younger than I had anticipated, her wavy blonde hair hanging loose around a delicate and pretty face. She was panting, and little beads of perspiration covered her forehead. "I sure am out of shape," she said, referring to the climb upstairs.

She addressed us as Mr. and Mrs. Alecson and took nothing for granted, including sitting before being offered a seat. If I'd felt a little sloppy before, I now felt downright slovenly before this well-dressed, well-mannered young lady. Perhaps, I mused, these truly irrelevant thoughts attested to a filament of vanity still glowing deep within.

We gave her a blow-by-blow description of what had occurred from my first pang of labor to the moment I was rushed into the operating room. She listened intently and took notes on a yellow legal pad. I told her about my morning phone conversation with Dr. Sherman and that we planned to meet with him and Dr. Pedro. She advised against that until we had counsel to represent us.

"Nancy," I said, "we are too curious not to have the meeting. We think Dr. Sherman is on our side and can help us understand what happened." I told Nancy that if Andrea's prognosis was hopeless, Lowell and I would want her to be taken off all life support and allowed to die.

Cautiously she said, "It would be better for the lawsuit that she should live."

"There's no way we're going to prolong her life for the sake of litigation," I stated.

Nancy left, saying that the senior partners of her firm would probably be interested in meeting with us. The concept of a malpractice lawsuit was utterly new to us, and we had no idea what it would involve. Our meeting with Nancy, a possible lawsuit—these were events on the periphery of our crisis.

We had our first real dinner, thanks to Doreen, and discussed various issues while consuming the casserole. Lowell's talk with my father and stepmother had made him more determined than ever to clarify the episodes leading up to Andrea's birth.

"I like Nancy," I said. "She seems genuinely to want to help us. What do you think of her?"

"I like her too, but I worry that she's too inexperienced. I would like to talk to some other lawyers before making a commitment." He was always a comparison shopper, whereas I grabbed whatever appealed to me first.

At noon the next day, we met with Drs. Sherman and Pedro. I immediately reminded Dr. Sherman of our phone conversation the previous morning. He said he didn't mean to imply that Dr. Kembel and June had been remiss in any way. He said everyone had acted as professionally as possible under the circumstances. His behavior was so sympathetic and kind that I found it impossible to pursue the matter. Instead, I asked him about Andrea.

"Mrs. Alecson, I feel there is hope for your daughter, which is what I told you at the hospital the day she was born. The normal sonogram, the fact that she was off the respirator within the first twenty-four hours and that the second seizure was brief, and from what I understand she hasn't had any seizures recently . . . these are all good signs. She could turn out fine."

"And what does 'fine' mean?" Lowell asked.

"It's not enough that she just be alive, you know. She has to have more than basic bodily functions," I interjected.

"Fine means more than basic bodily functions. Fine means normal."

Then I asked Dr. Pedro about the resuscitation. I wanted

to know if doctors always, automatically, resuscitate even if the baby has been without oxygen for a long time and if the baby has Apgar scores equal to or worse than Andrea's. Both doctors were taken aback.

"How could we not resuscitate? We didn't know how long she'd been without oxygen, and there was a heartbeat. Of course we'd resuscitate. What else would we do?" Dr. Pedro replied, in a tone of voice that suggested he had never had to answer such an outrageous question.

"The point I'm trying to make is, what if Andrea is not all right, wouldn't it have been better if she hadn't been resuscitated and had been allowed to die, as she would have, naturally, upon birth?"

They were nonplussed.

"Mrs. Alecson, your baby wasn't stillborn. How could we not resuscitate?" Dr. Sherman repeated.

I couldn't pursue this line of questioning any longer; I was on the verge of tears.

Dr. Sherman gave us a tour of the NICU, which was down the hall from the room where we were talking. He showed us around, speaking with great pride about the unit. He had the air of a public relations director as he tried to convince us to transfer Andrea back. I was so disarmed by his friendliness that I actually projected Andrea being there. The unit was smaller than the one Andrea was presently in, and I thought she might get more attention with Dr. Sherman in charge. When we parted, we told him we'd think about a transfer.

Boils had developed on my incision, yet I could not bring myself to see Dr. Kembel for an exam. I had called an obstetrician I had seen once, years ago when I needed a D & C, and made an appointment. So after the meeting, while Lowell went straight to visit Andrea, I headed back to the apartment for a rest, and then on to Dr. Gilmer's office.

When I sat down in Dr. Gilmer's examining room and she asked, "What can I do for you?" I began weeping uncontrollably. I tried to speak, but I couldn't. I thought, "This is it. I'm finally coming undone." She waited patiently until, between sobs, I told her I had just had a baby who was in intensive care. Looking at my incision, she said it was the cut of an emergency Caesarean. She displayed such disdain when I told her my primary caregiver was a midwife that I experienced profound regret that I hadn't used an obstetrician. She said she couldn't analyze what had happened because she'd need to see the records, but it seemed to her that things had not been handled right.

Lowell was home when I got back, heating up potatoes stuffed with crab meat—again, courtesy of Doreen. I went straight to bed to recuperate from an emotionally and physically exhausting day. I felt remorse that I hadn't made it to the NICU to see Andrea, but I just didn't have the strength for that in addition to the two appointments I'd had, which were miles apart.

As we ate dinner Lowell told me about his visit with Andrea. "When I got there, she was turned over on her stomach so her little fanny was exposed. The IV was still in her scalp, and they'd lowered the setting on the ventilator. They had tried lowering it last night, but she didn't like it, so they turned it back up. She trembles when I touch her. I rubbed her back lightly." His eyes began to fill with tears, and he took a deep breath. "Gloria put her little white booties on her." He was now sobbing, and we got up from the table to hold each other on the bed.

That evening, I wrote in my journal:

I have to have faith, which means storing my milk for her, seeing her, recognizing every little sign of progress. But I also must be able to let her go. How do I do both?

The closer I get, the more I bond and the more my maternal drive takes over. It is so difficult to maintain some neutral attachment. I either want to prepare myself for the worst by anticipating it—by imagining it—by holding back when I see her, or I want to completely indulge my love for this child who I carried for nine months. But when I let myself feel this love, I am overwhelmed by the pain, by the horrendous condition she is in. It seems too much to bear, and it's almost easier to lose hope. If I haven't any hope now, I won't grow close; I'll keep distant and I'll be able to accept the disappointment.

As was by now our custom, we called the NICU before going to sleep. We were told by the nurse that her phenobarbital level was at thirty and she was receiving a small amount for maintenance. Thirty was the magic number we had been waiting for.

4

Loss of Hope

When Lowell and I saw Andrea the next morning, eight days after her birth, she was what she had been all along: an exquisite doll under a spell. We took turns holding her, and we massaged her tender body. We kissed her fingers and toes, and we cried.

Dr. Hines spoke with us but did not venture a prognosis. However, he did give us the sense—restrained intimations—that there was brain damage. It didn't take special training in neonatology to figure that out. We could no longer blame the phenobarbital for her lack of response. The EEG was scheduled for that afternoon, and the CAT scan would be done after the weekend, on Monday.

"After the tests, we'll have the information we need to tell you more," he said, staring blankly at us.

"And when will there be results?" I asked.

"Hopefully, early next week."

I could have unloaded an avalanche of questions, ones I had ruminated over during these endless days, but I hadn't the heart. His body language said, "Please, do not ask me anything else. I cannot tell you anything else. I beg of you, leave me alone.'' This man seemed to me to have a better rapport with his tiny patients, who could not talk, respond, or trouble him with what they might think. His invalids, those "fetus-babies" as Lowell called them, did not ask questions.

We walked out of the hospital and stepped into a heat wave that was peaking. Summer in New York City was a season I usually wanted to escape. Sidewalks smoldered as forgotten refuse chemically transformed into a barrage of odors. Air thick with pollution and humidity stagnated in my lungs. This year, however, the discomforts of a summer suddenly upon us seemed nearly insignificant.

Holding hands, we walked to the bus. I had something on my mind to tell Lowell. It was difficult to say, for I had no idea how he'd react.

"Lowell, if we should lose Andrea, I would want to get pregnant as soon as I can."

"I would want that too," he replied.

"Oh God, Lowell, I didn't know what you'd say. I'm so grateful." I burst into tears and hugged him.

"I asked Dr. Gilmer, when she saw me the other day, about when I could conceive. She said by August. Of course, we have to see what happens." I thought, "Maybe we'd have a Skyler." Skyler was the name we had chosen for a boy child.

Did it lessen the pain to project into a future without Andrea, or with Andrea and another child? Did I really think I would have the spirit and the confidence to go on without Andrea, or with an incurably impaired Andrea—to go on and be pregnant again, to go through it all over again? During those moments when I could see a glimmer beyond the calamity engulfing me, I actually imagined the possibility of having what Lowell and I wanted: a healthy child. But these thoughts also made me feel uncomfortable and guilty of abandoning Andrea, if not in actuality, then in my mind.

I had no right to seek satisfaction for myself when her life was in limbo.

That evening, after Lowell put the air conditioner in the window and we picked at what was left of Doreen's stuffed potatoes (which deserved heartier appetites than ours), we were visited by Michelle, Lowell's friend from the Actor's Studio (where they were both members) and a sometime voice student of his. She brought us an assortment of foods that required little work to assemble into a meal. Although Lowell and I had always been fond of her, and were somewhat aware of events in her life, she was not a close friend. Yet I was moved by her willingness to step into our nightmare and witness what we were going through.

"Deborah," Michelle said, focusing her large, penetrating eyes on my face, "you don't look so bad. I thought you'd be paler. You look good."

"You think so?" I replied, unaware of how I looked since I hadn't studied my reflection in a mirror in more than a week, and barely recognized myself when I caught a glimpse.

Michelle made herself right at home, putting the perishables in our refrigerator. Among other edibles, she gave us a couple of cans of sardines—a surprising food, I thought—and she discussed ways of eating them. Then she talked about her own difficult birth experience with her now teenage son. She had also suffered the death of her young husband when her child was only three. Michelle was no stranger to loss, and I was beginning to see that people who have survived grief may be better able to acknowledge it in others. They know what to say and how to act, and they don't pretend that it doesn't exist.

"I would like to see the baby," Michelle said before leaving. I was bowled over. Lowell and she made plans to meet at the hospital on Monday.

In the evening, I called West-One.

"This is Mrs. Alecson. I believe Andrea had an EEG, and I was wondering if I can get the results."

"I'm sorry, but no one here knows what they are. You'll have to call after the weekend to talk with the attending," responded an unfamiliar voice.

"All right . . . I thought maybe . . . How is she?"

"Stable."

"Anything else?"

"No."

"Okay. Goodnight."

En route upstate to my father's house for a weekend of just the two of us, we stopped to see Andrea. Originally, when my father offered his home as a getaway while he and Kitty stayed at their studio in the city, I had felt unable to accept it. I was anxious about being seventy-five miles away from the hospital. But Lowell wanted to go, and my parents talked me into it.

"Deb, you need some distance," my father urged.

I yielded with the condition that we'd see Andrea before we left and immediately upon our return.

When we got to West-One, Gloria was towel-drying Andrea after having given her a bath. She was out of her isolette, and I was able to hold her while Lowell and I put baby lotion on her increasingly brittle skin. She wasn't tolerating the feedings, and she looked thinner. We both broke down, and Gloria held me as I cried.

"She's so sweet. Oh God . . . if only . . . ," I sobbed.

There was a time when I was inhibited and couldn't give into effusive emotions in public (except in the darkness of a theater). When I was with Andrea, I was incapable of suppressing them. I could not control my behavior, and I risked upsetting the many strangers who populated the NICU. Lowell, unlike every other man I had ever met in my life, was able to express his feelings: it was one of his strengths. But he had had to learn how. Acting classes, therapy, and his innate sensitivity were his teachers.

Gloria was comfortable around our emotional displays, and she'd do what came naturally: put her arm around our shoulders. That was all that was necessary.

"Gloria, we're going upstate for the weekend, so I want you to have the phone number. I'm a little nervous about being so far away."

"I think it's great that you're getting away. If anything should happen I will call you. You both should have some time together away from this place."

Why did I experience such remorse when redirecting my attention from Andrea to anything else?

My father's place in the country, which we called "The Farm" (it was a barn over a century old that he and my stepmother had converted), gave us the isolation and tranquillity we needed. Kitty had left a couple of club steaks in the refrigerator, and we picked up a bottle of Beaujolais in town. We dined outside on one of the patios, surrounded by lush foliage. Eating mostly in silence, we absorbed the natural world of grass, trees, and unobstructed sky. Birds perched on branches and rabbits skidding across the lawn made us feel as if we were seventy-five hundred miles away from the manmade world of West-One.

After dinner we went for a walk. Starting out, we came upon a baby doe nestled against the picket fence that edged the driveway. She looked up at us but did not stir; her face did not register fear.

"Lowell, do you think she's abandoned?"

"I don't know."

"Maybe she's hungry."

"What do they eat?"

"I'm not sure. She's a baby. I guess milk. I can give her

my breast milk. I can hold her in my lap and nurse her." I began to laugh.

"I suppose you can put some of your milk in a bowl and leave it by her face," Lowell suggested, also laughing.

"Well, let's see if she's still here when we get back."

She was, snuggled against the railing, as the sun set in a maroon sky that stretched all around us.

"Lowell, this is bizarre. Deer don't usually hang out right by the house like this. I feel as if this is a message from Andrea, but I don't know what it means."

We didn't want to get too close because of the risk of Lyme disease, but we were captivated. She was an innocent, like Andrea; and like Andrea, she had no mother there to protect her. We started to walk away, then I turned and approached her. Suddenly, she got up on her spindly legs and delicately strode into the brush.

The weekend in the country helped to remind me of the vagaries of nature. It brought to mind the saying "The Lord giveth, and the Lord taketh away," which I understood to mean that Andrea had her own fate, apart from mine.

Back in the city late on Monday morning, I got on the bus to go visit Andrea and, quite unexpectedly, found my mother aboard. We sat next to each other and talked. I told her about our weekend at The Farm and about my morning with Lowell.

"Lowell has been very upset, very angry, and taking it out on me. It wasn't until I started to cry that he snapped out of it and came to me."

"Did he talk?"

"He started to cry, and all he could say was 'It isn't fair.' "

"He's right. It isn't fair. Have you thought about seeing a therapist together?"

"Well, you know, he sees his therapist, and I had made

an appointment with Dr. Melner last week but had to cancel it when I saw the doctor about my incision. I'm to see him tomorrow. Maybe he can see me and Lowell at another time.''

''Or maybe he can recommend someone else.''

''Ma, I think Lowell and I have been handling everything really well. For the most part, we have been loving and responsive. But this is just the beginning. There are things that are going to come up, and it will help us sort out our feelings to have someone to talk to.''

''Absolutely,'' she agreed, giving me a hug.

My dear friend Enez was standing outside the NICU when we got there. The last time she and my mother had seen each other was at the baby shower. Ironically, it was Enez and her husband who got us *The New Child Health Encyclopedia* as a gift. I often looked through this book, rereading the section on asphyxia, while I pumped my breasts in Andrea's room. Enez was still recuperating from heart surgery she had had in December, and it was a physical effort, not to mention an emotional one, for her to make the subway trip from Brooklyn to visit Andrea. She had also learned that her heart valve, though supposedly fixed, was leaking, and more surgery was imminent.

''Enez, you didn't have to come. It's exerting. It's devastating. You're wonderful. Thank you.''

''Deborah, I took my time. Believe me, I did not race to get over here. I had to see your baby. I just had to. That's all there is to it. And I wanted to see you.''

My mother waited her turn to see Andrea while I ushered Enez into the nursery, first guiding her through the procedure of washing and wrapping in the paper gown.

Enez's eyes flooded instantly with tears as she looked at my sleeping beauty.

"Enez, I'm going to leave you for a minute because I see Dr. Hines, Andrea's primary doctor, and I have to talk to him."

Taking my mother, I followed Dr. Hines into his office and asked him if we could talk.

"What were the results of the CAT scan?" I asked.

"Mrs. Alecson, we weren't able to do it because the machine is down."

"The machine is down! There's only one machine in this entire hospital?"

"It's the one that we use for this unit."

"What does this mean?" I asked, on the brink of irrationality. There was something about Dr. Hines that seemed to elicit tantrums in me. Maybe it was the twenty milligrams of Valium I suspected were in his bloodstream, influencing his interpersonal relations. "Once it's fixed, Andrea will have the CAT scan," he answered in a calm, even voice.

"And how long will that take? Days, weeks, months?" I practically yelled.

"Mrs. Alecson, they are working on it now. We have a number of scans to do today."

"Dr. Hines, there is something I want you to know. If all the tests should indicate that Andrea's condition is as horrible and as terrible as we already suspect, we, that is to say Lowell and I and our families, including our parents, who are Andrea's grandparents, do not want her life prolonged. Do you understand? We cannot sentence her to the life of a vegetable. *Do you understand?*"

After a minute he responded, "Mrs. Alecson, I had heard that you felt this way from the nurses and practitioners, but this is the first time I've heard it directly from you."

"Okay, now you're hearing it from me. Can you please do everything in your power to make sure the CAT scan is done as soon as possible, and to have the results of that and the EEG made available?"

"I'll do my best. Once Dr. Maslin, the neurologist, has her report, we'll meet. That should be sometime this week."

The three of us sat in silence until I got up to leave. Though experience had proved otherwise, I somehow anticipated that Dr. Hines might say something I'd find significant.

Enez had to leave Andrea's side so that my mother could visit with her. She was just about speechless, which was unusual for my most talkative friend.

"Deb, if there's anything you need, if there's anything I can do, you know I'm here for you. You'll get through this. You and Lowell are strong. I love you."

That evening, Lowell's friend Richard came by, bearing pasta salad. They had met in summer stock years before. As a friend to Lowell, I had judged Richard to be lacking. He was, in my estimation, completely self-absorbed. It was uncanny how, when the three of us were together, Lowell or I might start talking about ourselves and within minutes be talking about Richard. I had always wished that Richard would be attentive, showing as much interest in Lowell as he showed in himself.

I was therefore thankful when I saw him embrace Lowell and hold him while Lowell cried. This time, we did not talk about Richard, and he was responsive to Lowell in a meaningful way.

During dinner Lowell told me that he had spoken to his friend Ben, who recommended that we talk to his father's lawyer.

"Deb, I would like to call this lawyer, Bruce Maxwell, and see what he has to say. Ben said, 'I know from experience he's one of the best, and you'll need that.' "

"But what about Nancy?" She had called back to tell us that her firm was interested in our case.

"I'm a little uneasy about her. She's young. This guy, Maxwell, is an older man, experienced. It can't hurt to meet him."

"Then I want to call Nancy and tell her."

Nancy sounded a little rejected, even hurt, when I told her that Lowell wanted to meet with other lawyers before making a decision.

"Is it because of my age? There are young lawyers in all firms," she said in her slow, careful way. Then she explained that she would only be assisting on the case and that one of the senior partners, whose specialty was medical malpractice, would be representing us. I relayed all this to Lowell, who still insisted on meeting Bruce Maxwell.

"Nancy, Lowell and I are new to lawyers, and he'll feel more comfortable choosing one after he has spoken to a few. Please understand. We're sure you are competent and can handle the case. We just need a little time."

She said she understood and would wait to hear from us. In the morning, Bruce Maxwell returned Lowell's call. I answered, and within seconds he had offended me. When he asked for Lowell, I said, "My husband's in the shower now, so I'll speak to you."

To which he replied, "It's good that he's clean."

I could not believe he would make so crude a comment.

I declared, "It's good that we get up in the morning and get out of bed and function"—and hung up.

When Lowell got out of the shower, I told him about my phone encounter. I did not want to meet the man, but I also did not want to oppose Lowell on this matter. He had tentatively arranged for Bruce Maxwell to come to our apartment the following evening to meet with us. Lowell agreed that the lawyer's response was pretty inappropriate, but he still wanted to have the meeting.

"Okay, but you'll have to call him back," I said, letting the issue drop.

I got to the hospital to find Andrea off the respirator. They had been lowering her settings all week, and she was adapting. We were scheduled to meet with Dr. Hines and the neurologist, Dr. Maslin, the next morning.

For the first time, I held Andrea in my arms without the foam mattress I had been using under her. The effort was rough on my back, but it felt so good to have her body touching mine. Gently, I wiped off the remains of the masking tape used to keep the mouthpiece of the respirator in place. When I finished, I realized that it was also the first time I was seeing her face in full. None of her features were covered. I thought, "God, she's cute. I believe she looks more like Lowell. She has his mouth."

While I had her in my arms, on my lap, I rubbed the delicate spot between her eyebrows, slightly above her nose. This place is known in Buddhist tradition as the "third eye" and is believed to emanate power. With the tip of my index finger I made circles, around and around, and spoke to her: "My sweet baby. You are so beautiful. I love you."

It was becoming more and more difficult to put her back in the isolette and leave the hospital. Could she possibly know, in the depths of her infant soul, that she was left behind?

I walked in a deluge from the hospital to Dr. Melner's office. He hugged me the minute I came through his door. I sat in that familiar chair across from him, feeling bewildered and mute. What could I say that might come close to describing what I felt?

Finally I began: "Every day I fall more in love with her. . . ."

At home, after the session, I was getting drunk on a second glass of wine, sitting on the couch, not answering the phone but watching as the machine recorded messages.

Lowell was at a friend's apartment giving voice lessons, and I expected him back soon with take-out food.

When he returned I was still on the couch, writing in my journal: "Her being off the respirator—is this a blessing or a curse?"

Over dinner, we discussed the events of our day. I told Lowell about my session. "Melner spoke about his ex-wife. Their first child was a stillbirth. She went on to have another child the following year. He said our situation was bringing it all back, and he was concerned that it would affect his work with me. So we decided to see how it goes. He's leaving on vacation soon anyway, and in the meantime he's recommended a woman therapist who, because of a personal tragedy, is especially good with parents and couples. Maybe we can see her together at some point."

"Yes, I would be willing. You know, it seems the more people we talk to about Andrea, the more stories we hear."

It was true. So many of the people we spoke to had had disasters of their own, or knew of people who had nearly died in childbirth, or had a baby with severe anomalies, or were themselves compensating for deficits caused by fetal distress or the trauma of birth. It seemed more women had Caesareans than experienced natural childbirth; there always was some complication, be it major or minor.

The word from West-One, before Lowell and I retired, was that Andrea was stable but less active. I finally fell asleep after hours of lying there thinking about what "less active" could signify and what our alternatives were given all the negative and positive results the doctors might report.

The next morning was our meeting at the hospital. Dr. Hines, Dr. Maslin, Dr. Miron (the fellow), and Enid, the nurse practitioner, invited Lowell and me into a large room where we could talk. We sat down with pads and pens, ready to take notes. They were all in obvious discomfort as they struggled to get the meeting under way. I could tell that Dr. Maslin was groping to find the right words. She started by referring to the outcome of the tests rather than to Andrea's condition. She spoke about Andrea's brain as if it were something separate from Andrea herself. I jotted down: "CAT very abnormal, decreased oxygen, dark cortex, stroke, hemorrhage into the thalamus (relay station), brain stem looks normal (why she can breathe on her own), severe damage to *both* hemispheres; EEG—there's some activity but very abnormal, simple as opposed to rich, always some activity vs. spurts then none. . . ."

I was reeling from the medical terms, and the challenge to understand what they meant kept my emotions in check. Dr. Maslin concluded, "It's hard to tell you exactly how she'll do." I could not believe my ears. How hard could it possibly be? We weren't concerned about whether Andrea would one day master trigonometry. We were concerned about whether she would ever open her eyes and become aware of herself as a human being. We were concerned that her life would be continually wracked by seizures—meaning that she'd have to be medicated to the point of sedation.

I unleashed a torrent: "Will she ever suck and have any normal reflexes? Will she sit up, roll over, creep, crawl, walk, speak? Will she ever recognize me as her momma? Will she experience any pleasure or interaction with life? Will she ever be able to do more than lie in bed, oblivious to the world?"

My emotions were taking over, and I heard my voice becoming strained. Dr. Hines talked about the one-in-a-billion baby who grows up "to function"—minimally, but still, function.

"Functioning is not enough," I interrupted.

Dr. Maslin grew bold and made a projection for Andrea:

"She would probably be moderately to severely developmentally delayed, and she'd need physical therapy. As far as whether she'll be aware of you, I cannot say."

From the sound of it, they believed that she would survive. Dr. Hines said, "We'd repeat the EEG and MRI (magnetic resonance imaging) when she's older. In a month or two." Then there was the BAER (brain stem auditory evoke response) test they were to do later in the day, to test for hearing impairment.

I thought with alarm, "When she's older?"

Lowell studied the CAT scan negative as Dr. Maslin pointed out bright spots and dark spots. What was more surprising to me than the outcome of the tests was the reluctance, as it seemed to me, of these medical professionals to convert the data into behavioral expectations. If these people couldn't, who could? No one would utter aloud what everyone in that room knew without a shadow of a doubt: as a human being, Andrea was fated to an existence of utter impoverishment. Her condition was irreversible, this much was clear; the damage could never be undone.

Before the meeting ended and the doctors went on with their duties, I felt an urgent need to pronounce, once again, our wishes for Andrea, particularly in light of this latest information. I demanded their attention and began my speech: "I have been a special educator for years, and I know the possibilities and options for handicapped children in this society. But we're not even talking about 'handicapped' with Andrea; we're talking about the complete annihilation of a person, with no hope of having any of the most basic qualities that make us human and make life worth living. Lowell and I and both our families have discussed this, and we do not want Andrea's life to be prolonged. There is no point. It would not be in her best interest or in ours, and we have to go on with our lives. So I'm asking you, what can be done?"

These professionals were used to seeing parents enter a state of shock and mental incapacitation upon hearing such a bleak prognosis. My request for action clearly disarmed them. They probably thought the hard part—giving us the news—was over.

Dr. Hines said, "You can sign a DNR—a Do Not Resuscitate order—to keep her off of the respirator. That should not be problematic."

"But she's not on the respirator," Lowell pointed out.

"Well, a DNR will keep her off, just in case."

"Okay, what else?" I asked.

"There is nothing else," Dr. Hines replied.

"What about the IV and feeding tube? She's not able to suck, and she'll never be able to feed herself," I said, not knowing where I was going with this.

"We can't withhold nutrition and hydration," he said emphatically.

"But she can go on forever like this, right? *Something* has to be done." I beseeched everyone in the room.

Dr. Hines remained behind after the others had left. He told us about the existence of an ethics committee at the hospital, which could convene on our behalf to discuss Andrea and our wishes for her.

"Will Lowell and I be at that meeting?"

"Probably not. We need to talk among ourselves first."

I was feeling too shattered to argue.

Then, in his own faltering way, he let us know that he was on our side, as were the others, but there were restrictions. We'd have to take it one step at a time.

We visited with Andrea and took turns holding her. She got the hiccups in my arms, and I was reminded of all the times she'd had the hiccups in my womb. She was congested, and her breathing was labored. She was moving less.

Gloria came around to suction her. "I suppose you know the results of the tests," I said. She nodded. "Dr. Hines is going to see about getting the ethics committee to meet. You know how Lowell and I feel. We can't let Andrea continue this way.'' She continued to nod her head while settling Andrea on her mattress.

"Gloria, do you agree with us? Do you agree that if she should live it would be awful?''

"In her case, yes. And I hope that the committee goes with you. But I have seen a child in a condition similar to Andrea's kept on life support after the parents made the same request as yours. So please, understand that what you want for your daughter may be impossible. I don't know what else to say. We all know how you feel.'' Then she closed the lid of the isolette.

At home we pulled ourselves together before our meeting with Bruce Maxwell at the Atrium Club. I had said that I didn't want to meet him, so Lowell left word with his secretary to call before coming over. Maxwell called back and admitted to Lowell that he and I had "got off to a bad start.'' He said he'd like to treat us to dinner. Lowell really wanted me to come along, so I acquiesced, figuring that I'd at least get a decent meal.

"You know, Lowell, it occurs to me that our potential case could be worth a lot of money to some lucky lawyer,'' I said as I looked for something to wear.

"Of course, Deb,'' Lowell replied, having come to the same conclusion.

I found an old standby dress in my closet that I hadn't worn since pre-pregnancy, and it actually fit. I had lost all my pregnancy weight in less than two weeks! There's nothing like trauma to keep one in shape.

We were to meet Maxwell at the bar of this fancy establishment on the Upper East Side. While waiting we ordered a glass of wine each, which for us was an indulgence. We had become painfully aware of our finances now that the medical bills were starting to appear in our mailbox. Insurance would pay for my stay at the hospital, but we weren't sure how much of Andrea's care—a minimum of one thousand dollars a day, not including doctor fees—would be covered.

Maxwell arrived late, together with his assistant, Carol, an attractive woman in her late forties. He apologized for the delay, blaming it on the traffic. Maxwell was a large man with a full voice who seemed to be in the habit of impressing people. As we sat down at "his" table, he greeted the maitre d', waitresses, and waiters with warm familiarity and ordered a round of drinks for us all. I declined, wanting to remain as sober as possible. Maxwell and Carol struck me as the old-fashioned team of the male boss who wheels and deals and his ever-faithful female assistant who keeps things running smoothly in business and private affairs alike, remembering his wedding anniversary for him and shopping for gifts for the wife. I did not want to like this man.

Suddenly I was overcome by a delayed reaction to the earlier meeting with the doctors, combined with a resistance to discussing my baby's catastrophic birth in lawyer-ese. Unable to eat my food or make small talk with Maxwell and Carol, much less discuss Andrea by candlelight, I bolted from my seat, mumbling an excuse as tears rolled down my face. Not knowing where to go, I ended up in a stall in the women's bathroom, where I sat on the toilet seat and wailed. Every so often a customer would step into the bathroom and tentatively use the facility after inquiring, "Are you all right?" over the partition. It was as if in one instant the enormity of my grief seized me and I was paralyzed with despair. I did not think I could stop crying or ever move from that toilet seat.

Eventually Carol came to find me. She coaxed me out of the stall, and as I leaned against a sink, patting my swollen eyes with a wet paper towel, she expressed genuine sorrow over what had happened. She wasn't latching on to a big case now; she was just being compassionate. I returned to the table, with Carol leading the way. Since I was clearly in no shape to continue the meal or the meeting, Lowell and I grabbed a cab and went home.

At ten-thirty that evening, Lowell spoke with a nurse on West-One. I looked over his shoulder as he wrote in the notebook we were keeping on Andrea: "feeding—5 cc's every 2 hours (seems to be tolerating the feeding); still breathing on her own—nurse exercises her arms and they seem to tense up."

Before going to bed, I wrote:

> Though I sobbed while holding Andrea, I felt less the im-
> pulse of attachment and more the beginnings of letting go.
> We have set in motion the process of freeing her soul.
> Now all my prayers are for the ethics committee to bend
> to our wishes and not fight us.

I fell asleep having not pumped my breasts. I planned to stop cold turkey. It was my act of renunciation.

When I awoke the next morning, I could not move; the pain radiating from my breasts was so intense that I nearly blacked out when I tried to sit up. My breasts felt like slabs of stone weighing on my chest. I called Dr. Gilmer, who advised that I wear an ace bandage wrapped tightly around my bosom, use ice packs, and take milk of magnesia.

As fate would have it, my oldest friend in the world, Becky, whom I had met in a Brooklyn kindergarten class and who had been living for years in California, was in New York. We hadn't seen each other in five years, though we kept up a constant correspondence by mail and never missed a birthday phone call. I had expected a visit from her sometime that summer, and I had written to her when I was in the hospital to prepare her for the blow. She called me after she had settled in at a mutual friend's in New York, sounding chirpy and ecstatic to meet the new Alecson.

"Becky, you never got my letter?"

"What letter?"

When she came to our apartment, she found me in bed, dressed in a nightshirt and my flannel robe, under two blankets and a comforter, my teeth chattering in my head. The engorgement had caused a fever. Becky was a masseuse, and she started right away to massage my feet. We passed the morning talking, catching up on each other's lives, and refilling the packs with ice cubes. I was alone when Dr. Hines called to tell us that the DNR was ready to be signed and that the ethics committee would meet Monday morning, without us.

"Dr. Hines, it is extremely important to me that the members of the ethics committee see Andrea with their own eyes and that she doesn't remain a case or statistic or summation of tests."

"I understand, Mrs. Alecson. Dr. Maslin will be on the committee, as well as others who are personally involved with your daughter. So when can I expect you to sign the order?"

Quite uncharacteristically, I was embarrassed to explain to the doctor why I would not be able to race over to the hospital that instant. I felt shy just talking to him on the phone from my bed! Finally I simply told him, "I'm a little out of sorts right now. I've stopped pumping my breast milk and I am engorged. I can't imagine how I could make it to the hospital today when I can barely make it to the next room."

We decided that Lowell would meet with him at seven that evening.

Then Dr. Kembel called, having received my earlier message. He and June were the only ones who could tell me what kind of incision I had inside, since the external one ran vertically and a next pregnancy would be somewhat risky if the internal cut was vertical as well. He said it was transverse, which was what I wanted to hear. Then he asked about Andrea and about my health.

"Presently, I am suffering with engorged breasts."

"Use ice."

"I am. Okay, thanks for getting back to me."

He never asked me why I hadn't seen him for a postoperative exam.

I lay in bed and thought that I didn't hate June or Dr. Kembel, unless unconsciously. I closed my eyes and I could see Andrea's face so clearly—her little open mouth and her delicate nostrils. My father had said we would need to think of alternatives in case the ethics committee turned us down. I told him, "I'll abduct her, take her home, and let her die in my arms." He replied, "Yes and no."

Never during my nine blissful months of pregnancy could I have imagined that I might one day want the death of my baby.

That afternoon I spoke with Dr. Eric Cassell, a well-known and highly regarded ethicist and medical doctor. His name was given to me by my parents, who knew someone who knew him and recommended that I speak with him. I was nervous calling him because of his stature in the medical field and because I did not know if he'd be sympathetic to our wishes for Andrea. It was heartening when, without the usual fuss of doctors in busy offices, he took my call right away. After introductions, he mentioned a phone conversation he had had with my stepmother and said he was expecting to hear from me. I summarized our situation, which he grasped immediately. To my relief, he did not judge us; instead he listened, generously, to what I had to say. He focused on the mindset I should have regarding the ethics committee, on the kind of attitude I should exhibit. "It is important that you do not put them on the defensive. You do not want to become adversaries. You should acknowledge their concern for your baby's welfare. Remember, you are making a gentle request for help." Then he gave me the name of a pediatrician and fellow at the Hastings Center (for bioethical research), Dr. Kathy Nolan.

Dr. Nolan was almost tender in her conversation with me, and completely supportive of our position. Regarding the ethics committee and their decision, she said, "It's going to take a few days. They're going to size you up." She stressed that we had to make them aware of our beliefs concerning the quality of life and our understanding that our child would never be able to function as a member of society. She would never learn, and she might not survive. "You must say that you think it is cruel to keep her alive by forced feedings." She assured me that I should feel free to call her and that she would try to help us as best she could. I felt an instant rapport with her and knew that Andrea, Lowell, and I had just made a friend.

That evening, Lowell returned the breast pump to the pharmacy, then went to the hospital to sign the DNR. He learned from Dr. Hines that the BAER test was also abnormal—something about a wave of five when one and three are within normal range. He stayed with Andrea for a couple of hours and spoke with her caregiver, Susan. Susan told Lowell that Andrea was not responsive and not retaining food: "She is the most unresponsive I have ever seen her."

I went to sleep wondering if Andrea knew, in some mystical way, that we wanted her to let go and die.

Gradually, over the weekend, my breasts began to soften, and I went for my first swim in the pool. If I could have gone incognito, I would have. When I was last in a bathing suit, it was the day before I went into labor, and Andrea went swimming too. I could not bear the prospect of running into acquaintances who would observe the absence of a belly and ask cheerful questions. I managed to slip through the locker room unnoticed, but the lifeguard stopped me to hear the good news. All I could say was, "I had a disaster"; he blanched and replied, "I'm sorry."

Saturday night I completely dissolved. The greatest source of my distress was knowing that Andrea scarcely got touched or held when we weren't there with her. If she had been able to suck, she would have been held for at least the length of time it took to drink a bottle. The unit was often understaffed, and caressing the infants was superfluous. I couldn't shake the image of her adrift in space, cut off from all human contact. Of course, I also knew that she probably couldn't tell if she was being held anyway. Here I was trying to convince the hospital to let her die while agonizing over the lack of attention she received. It was all so senseless.

I ran into Leona the next day at the health club. We hadn't spoken since my release from the hospital. I was disappointed that she hadn't called to find out how we all were, but I didn't mention that. Instead I told her about my current obsession that Andrea be touched and held by the nursing staff. She suggested that I ask one of the nurses to put a note on her isolette saying, "Hold me," or some such thing.

That evening I wrote:

Tomorrow the ethics committee meets without us. I asked Dr. Hines what's ethical about the committee, and he didn't understand my question. When I think of her life prolonged, I cannot bear it. I love her so much. She remains so sweet and beautiful. Her little legs are perpetually folded tight like chicken wings. Her hands quiver at any movement or sudden touch. Susan lifted her eyelids today and I saw her eyes: Lowell's color. Lowell and I took turns holding her, and we extended her limbs and spread baby lotion on her skin.

Monday morning, Lowell went to work and I went to the hospital. I wanted to be there when the meeting ended so that I could learn of the outcome. I sat with Andrea on my lap, stroking her head, and said, ''Soon we will know if you will be set free.'' I spotted Gloria and Enid across the rows of isolettes and beckoned them to me.

For Lowell

Our love fused in my womb grew
as microscopic matter and
the imaginings of our minds.

First months like motion sickness
followed by calm
then helium belly that bulged
with creature kicks
until the being had a sex, then name,
and we called her Andrea.

We prepared her place on earth:
toys shelved in greeting,
drawers filled with soon-to-be belongings,
an empty cradle rocked in anticipation.

We labored for two days
and still she couldn't budge,
stuck in the canal facing
her own peculiar direction.

An emergency too late
pulled her blue from my body.

Our little girl lies silent
staring in a place we never prepared,
with a tube threaded through her throat
to keep her alive when dead to the world.

5

A Decision Reversed

"What was decided?" I asked, looking up at Gloria and Enid, holding Andrea on my lap, swaddled in a blanket.

They glanced at each other, as if seeking permission to speak.

"They are all in agreement with you. It was unanimous," Gloria exclaimed, her eyes clouding with tears.

"Oh God, I can't believe it." I started to cry. "But what does this mean? What are they agreeing to?"

"We can't really tell you more. The committee will meet with you and Lowell tomorrow afternoon," Gloria replied.

I could not wait until tomorrow.

I saw that they were struggling to be tactful without being blatant because it was the responsibility of Dr. Hines and the head of the department, Dr. Stein, to inform us of the consensus of the group.

"Gloria, Enid, I beg of you, what was decided?"

Again, they turned to each other.

"They agree, we agree, that it would be best for Andrea that she be allowed to die," Gloria affirmed.

"But, they need to come up with the most humane and compassionate way," Enid interjected.

I was dumbfounded.

"And the feedings?" I asked.

"They are considering your request to withhold feeding and the IV, and they are also looking into other ways," Gloria said.

"How long would that take, if the feedings stop? How long would it take for her to die?" I asked, even as I thought, "Is this really happening? Am I having this conversation?"

Enid answered, "Two to three weeks."

"Would she be uncomfortable, in pain?"

"No. She'd probably be given sugar water, and in her condition, with her neurological damage, she wouldn't suffer."

"I can't believe it, I just can't believe it. It's unbelievable that they are going to help us." I was overcome by a feeling of unreality.

I shifted Andrea in my arms, hugging her to my chest. Her eyes were closed, and her mouth hung open.

Gloria asked if I was all right and if I wanted her to put Andrea back in the isolette.

"I'm okay. I want to hold her. I'll call you when I'm ready to go. I just need to be with her now."

Brushing the back of my hand across her cheek, I spoke to her: "My precious, precious baby, there will be an end to your suffering . . . to mine . . . your father's. We will be with you and make sure you are comfortable. This is the only thing I can do for you. And maybe you'll be born again, healthy and whole. I love you so much. I'm sorry. Oh God, I am so sorry."

I sat still for a few minutes, staring through the windows at the mercurial water of the river beyond, shining dully in the afternoon sunlight. It was a view I had grown accustomed to gazing upon. When I needed privacy, I would turn my back on the frenzy of the NICU and sob while absorbing the unceasing motion of the waterway below. I would think of the wisdom gleaned through the ages from watching water, in its innumerable guises, flow. With Andrea behind me, alive but not living, lying prostrate in her isolette, I would search the river for answers. Why Andrea? Why me? How do I accept that which is not in my control?

I had a date with Sheila for a glass of wine at O'Neals, a pub and restaurant near Lincoln Center. When I got there I went directly to the public phone to call my mother.

"Ma, I spoke with Gloria and Enid after the committee met. They've decided to go with us, to let her die."

She started to cry, but I couldn't tell if it was from relief or regret. Then she told me that my grandparents had been in an accident aboard a city bus in Brooklyn, and they were both in the hospital. My grandmother had broken her hip; my grandfather had been knocked unconscious, though he had since come to.

"My God. This is too much. They'll be all right, won't they?"

She planned to visit them that evening and would have a better idea of the situation then. My aunt and uncle, her siblings, were already involved. Then she asked, "Did you say goodbye to Andrea?"

"No, I'm going to be with her until the end."

When I got to the bar I found Sheila perched on a stool. Over drinks, I told her of the latest family disaster and discussed the decision of the ethics committee.

"Sheil, there are no words in the English language to describe the mixture of feelings I experienced when I heard that Andrea's death is imminent. I was holding her, comforting her. I can't believe that the torture will be over, that she'll be set free. Now at last I'll be able to start letting go and to prepare myself for her death.''

''Well, I guess this is good news. Good news, bad news, it's hard to tell which is which. Have you told Lowell?''

''He had his first day back at the high school, then he had an appointment to see his therapist, so by the time I get home he should be there. It's all just, I don't know . . .''

I was sitting on the couch when Lowell walked in the door. He was a few feet into the apartment when I burst out with the news: ''Lowell, they're going to let her die.''

He sat down beside me, and we hugged each other and cried.

''I can't believe it,'' he said. ''I can't believe it. Thank God. Are you sure?''

I told him about my conversation with Gloria and Enid and how they said it should take two to three weeks.

''They'll make sure she's comfortable, not suffering. There's more that has to be worked out. We're to meet with them tomorrow.'' We talked about my grandparents, who, according to a phone message from my mother, were not in critical condition and were being well taken care of at the hospital. I planned to call them after dinner.

Lowell's supervisor at work, Steve, had taken him aside to talk, to learn of Andrea's condition, and to comfort him. ''Steve told me about someone he knew from his church whose child was severely damaged at birth and had to be carried around in a basket.''

The image of a child being lugged around in a basket struck me as absurd, and I became hysterical, first with laughter, then with tears. What kind of life was that?

Lowell and I went to bed that evening gripped by emotions we had never felt before: gratefulness intertwined with sadness, a burdened relief.

First thing next morning, a nurse named Martina answered the phone at West-One and reported that Andrea was "doing pretty good" but not tolerating the feedings, so she was receiving hyperalimentation (the IV).

We stopped in on Andrea before meeting with Dr. Stein and some of the others from the ethics committee. It was a brief visit that reaffirmed our conviction to let her go. Andrea was a corporeal presence whose chest rose and fell as if feigning life. She had been dying since birth.

The mood was tense and funereal as we took our seats in Dr. Stein's office, forming a loose circle with Gloria, Enid, the social worker, and Dr. Hines. Lowell and I sat side by side, holding hands, waiting for Dr. Stein—whom we were meeting for the first time—to tell us what we had already learned from Gloria and Enid.

Dr. Stein, an austere man of intimidating detachment, began the meeting by reporting in a monotone that the ethics committee had met to discuss a course of treatment for our daughter. Then, in a single compact sentence, offered almost as an aside, he declared that our request to withhold nutrition must be denied.

I turned to look at Gloria, whose face expressed utter surprise. I lost my power of speech as I experienced vertigo and grasped onto the arms of the chair to keep upright. I had never felt so betrayed in all my life.

He continued talking about "appropriate treatment in light of Andrea's condition" (he acknowledged her damage to be irreversible), but I was no longer listening. The only thing that registered was that the one and only means by which Andrea could have peacefully died was refused her. She was sentenced to exist: in her case, a fate worse than death.

"With the feedings continued, how long can she go on?" I asked the group, my voice shaking.

No one could say exactly; I heard conjectures of months, possibly years—into adolescence, young adulthood.

Dr. Stein was droning on about the misfortune of our situation and the responsibility of the hospital to "provide a minimal level of care."

Interrupting him, I declared, "What you are saying is you agree with us that Andrea should be allowed to die but there is nothing you can do about it."

"Yes," he replied.

"How about releasing her into our custody?" Lowell asked.

"We can't do that because we are aware of your intentions," Dr. Stein answered.

"She's no longer our baby. She's your baby," I said. The truth of my statement resounded throughout my being. I unearthed an involuntary high-pitched scream, then ran from the room.

Once again, I found myself in a public bathroom sitting on a toilet seat, out of my mind. This time I had completely regressed; I felt like a helpless child who could not get a cruel adult to do what I so desperately wanted. My state and circumstance reminded me of an experience I'd had at a family gathering when I was a child. I had accidentally locked myself in the bathroom of my grandparents' apartment, and the local fire department had to be called to rescue me. My predicament was made all the more demeaning by my mother's brother, who cracked jokes while stuffing an endless number of playing cards under the door at me. I had felt frightened and powerless and, thanks to my uncle, shamed as well.

There I was, four years old again: scared, weak, and humiliated. Lowell was knocking on the door, calling, "Honey, it's me. Let me in."

Peeking my head cautiously out the door, somehow expecting hospital security to be lying in wait, I led him into the bathroom. In his arms I repeated, "How are we going to survive this? How will I live? This is so terrible."

Several minutes passed before I was able to leave the sanctuary of the bathroom. In the hallway were Gloria and Enid, who rushed to my side, terribly upset.

"Oh Deborah, we didn't know Dr. Stein would change his mind. We were as shocked as you. Something must have happened. I'm so sorry," Gloria exclaimed.

I was trying to hold back, to be steady and lucid, to accept what they were saying. Then either Gloria or Enid mentioned something about the hospital lawyers. I heard it hazily, as if it was uttered at a great distance from me. All I could do was embrace Gloria and Enid, and for an instant we three stood with arms wrapped around one another. From the corner of my eye I saw Dr. Stein and the others in the hallway, outside Stein's office. I worried that he might perceive such a demonstration by Gloria and Enid as unprofessional and untrustworthy.

"We'll call later," I promised Gloria as Lowell and I headed for the elevators.

Lowell had to lead me out of the hospital and along the street with a hand under my elbow. It was as if my volition had been obliterated. He steered me down steps, onto subway platforms, and into trains, until we reached the offices of Schwartz, McKensey, and Pagan, attorneys at law— Nancy Cronin's firm, where we had an appointment.

We were buzzed into what appeared to be a fortress housed in a brownstone. The entryway and staircases, with balustrades of polished brass, were of white marble. An elevator encased in black wrought iron brought us to the upper level, the reception area. We were told to have a seat in a waiting room of harshly modern decor that was separated by glass from the inner sanctum, where young men and women manned the phones, answered the intercoms, and monitored the clients.

"Lowell, I don't know how I'm going to handle this," I said, checking my reflection in the glass of a grotesque painting that hung above the couch.

"You'll be all right," he said as he straightened his tie.

At last we were summoned. We took the elevator to David Schwartz's office, an enormous room, sumptuously furnished, that was probably the size of our entire apartment. Schwartz, a rather good-looking man in his early forties, who had the body shape of someone who worked long hours at a desk and ate gourmet delicacies too soon before bed, bid us welcome. It was soon obvious to him that I was in some sort of shock, and he offered me a drink, which I readily accepted. He had a full bar, complete with crystal glasses that reminded me of the unreality of the movies. I expected Cary Grant to pop up and offer me a cigarette from an eighteen-carat gold case.

Schwartz wanted his partner, Ricky Pagan, to join us, so we contained ourselves before launching into our story. Pagan arrived, a man quite a bit less dapper than Schwartz, bordering on disheveled. He loomed over us all; I imagined him on a basketball court at an Ivy League college somewhere, once upon a time.

We explained that we had just come from a meeting with some members of the hospital's ethics committee and were stunned by a reversal of decision regarding Andrea. As our lawyers, I knew, they could not be in accord with our wish that Andrea be allowed to die. If indeed malpractice could be established, it would only be to everyone's monetary advantage that she be kept alive.

I sat in a daze, listening to Lowell describe my labor and the birth, occasionally offering a detail or a clarification. I watched Schwartz and Pagan to see if they exhibited com-

passion for our situation. I didn't need their sympathy, but
I did need to feel that they would handle our grievance with
something other than dollar signs in their eyes. Pagan, who
would be the one to represent us, said, "I think you have
liability here. You went into the hospital pregnant and
healthy, and this terrible thing happened to your daughter.
It looks to me like the result of some negligence."

They could not tell us more, they said, until they saw the
records, which would have to be reviewed by their medical
experts.

Lowell, extending his hand, said, "Thank you for your
time. Deborah and I need to talk, then we'll be in touch
with you."

Waiting for the elevator to take us to the street, I asked
Lowell, "So, what do you think?"

"They seem knowledgeable, and they seem to think we
have a case. We need to discuss it more. What do you
think?"

"Well, you know I like Nancy, and she'd be involved if we
used them. They appeared genuinely moved, would like to
see some justice done, some compensation. Judging by their
offices, they must have won a number of cases. I'm too out
of it now to think more clearly."

It was past dinnertime. We wandered around the neighborhood looking for an affordable restaurant, then finally
decided to go back to the apartment and order a pizza for
the third time that week. Hospital bills were pouring in, and
we could not bring ourselves to spend frivolously—which
included a meal out.

In fact, when we arrived home we were greeted by a bill
that had become a persistent annoyance: a Dr. Henry,
whom we never heard of, claimed to have done something
to or something for Andrea that cost $341. This weekly
bill—one among many—felt like some, as yet undefined,

form of harassment. It also represented the injustice of having a hospital keep our daughter alive against our wishes, and having to pay for the expense of doing so.

Before going to West-One in the morning, I called Dr. Cassell to tell him about the reversal of the decision and to ask for advice on how best to proceed. He sounded already aware of what was going on.

"I think Dr. Stein is wrong," he said. What a relief it was to hear him say that.

"There is internal dissension, and they haven't resolved what to do about it," he assured me. "The lawyers for the hospital have reviewed the situation and are concerned about legal implications." Talking to him was like talking to the Wizard of Oz. I had yet to meet him face to face, but I endowed him with the power to right wrongs and to convince all concerned to give Andrea what she was entitled to: a merciful death.

He said the issue of withholding nutrition was particularly thorny because of the "Baby Doe" case. I recalled Dr. Stein saying something about Baby Doe regulations.

He concluded with the advice, "Wait. Be patient. And don't push the hospital group."

When I got off the phone, I set myself a task: to investigate legal cases that might be influencing the hospital administrators. Just who was Baby Doe?

I spoke with Kathy Nolan, who tried to explain the legal intricacies of withholding nutrition. I didn't understand why it was no big deal to get a DNR, but impossible to stop the feedings Andrea was continually rejecting. Why was it acceptable to deny her a respirator if her breathing should fail but unacceptable to stop artificial feedings? After all, they both resulted in death. I was confused. It didn't make sense.

Dr. Nolan said that the federal government (as specified in the Baby Doe Regulations of 1983) considered giving food to be "customary medical care"—ordinary, appropriate treatment—whereas withholding nutrition from impaired newborns was deemed to be child abuse and neglect. "The real question, though, is whether it is appropriate to feed a baby who will never be able to feed herself and whose long-term prognosis is like Andrea's," she said. "There's a case in Missouri, the Cruzan case. This family has been trying to get the feeding tube removed from their comatose daughter who has been in a vegetative state for six years. The courts have to decide whether giving her food and water is heroic treatment or simply basic care. Without the feeding tube she would starve to death, and so removing it can be perceived as euthanasia, which is illegal in this country. We have to watch this case closely, for it has direct bearing on your situation with Andrea," she concluded.

I had a lot to learn—about Baby Doe, the Cruzan case, and euthanasia. All I knew so far was that the Baby Doe case began in 1982, when a baby born in Indiana with multiple birth defects was allowed to die in the hospital. The story of this baby, Baby Doe, had a direct bearing on the fate of my own baby.

When I arrived at the hospital I found Andrea on her belly, legs splayed like a frog's, the IV inserted in her left leg and a nasogastric tube threaded into her left nostril. Mom was there already. We spoke with Dr. Hines, who said Dr. Stein had ordered the feeding tube, which would now be pretty much a permanent fixture. Enid was also present; she added, "The hope is to get her off the IV, but it probably won't work. She'll vomit the food up."

I winced and thought, "Don't they see that she wants to die? How can they pour food down her nose when her body rejects it? Oh God, it's so cruel. It's an assault."

Standing over Andrea's isolette, my mother and I talked.

"Mom, you know she can go on and on like this. Do you think you're going to continue coming here to see her?"

"I don't know, honey."

"I don't know either. I mean, I haven't given up. Lowell and I have talked about trying to get her transferred to another hospital or a hospice. Then there's legal action to consider."

"Deb, maybe it would do you good to get away for a while, to stop obsessing."

"You think I'm obsessing?"

"I think you need to step back a little. To take a breather."

"I can't."

At home, Lowell was giving a voice lesson. We were expecting Becky to come by soon and prepare dinner for everyone. She had been spending her days visiting her New York friends and going to her favorite haunts. When we last spoke, she had asked about Andrea: "Would you love her if she was in an institution?" I told her I couldn't think about that. "You could visit her," she said. I had asked Becky if she would come with me to see Andrea, but she said she couldn't handle it. When we were kids, already best friends, her older brother had been murdered. From out of the blue, without even robbery as a motive, a gang of teenagers had knifed him as he was walking along a street in the Bronx. I always felt that Becky had never really dealt with that unfathomable loss and with the capriciousness of death. As an adult, she was still running from that pain, so I understood her inability to witness the tragedy of Andrea.

As I sat outside our bedroom/music room, listening to Jackie, a voice student, sing scales within, I felt a despair come over me that I could not ward off. Pouring myself a large glass of white wine, I went into the nursery where I could close the louvered doors and be alone. Becky was late, the voice lesson was coming to an end, and I could not face anyone, including Lowell. I wanted to disappear.

Curled in fetal position under a blanket on the linoleum floor of the nursery, I imagined killing Andrea myself. How would I do it? I'd hold my hand over her mouth. When the police came to arrest me, I'd plead insanity compounded by postpartum depression. Surely the court would take mercy on me. But what if they didn't? I couldn't let myself be locked away, away from Lowell. It would be too awful for him to live with. I thought, "If I wasn't with Lowell, I would kill her. If I was alone in this, I would have nothing to lose."

As if miles away, I heard Jackie and Lowell conversing in the kitchen, their voices muffled; then the front door slammed. Lowell approached the nursery and said, "Deb, are you in there? Are you all right?" His voice stunned me as I lay, transfixed, staring into space. With Herculean effort, I responded: "I need to be by myself."

The buzzer rang, and Lowell let Becky into the apartment. They talked, barely audible; I figured that Lowell was telling Becky that I was in a state. I heard a rustling noise that I assumed was grocery bags being unpacked, and the clanging of pots on the stove. I could not move from my spot on the floor. I felt suspended in time.

The two of them gently opened the louvered doors and asked me to come join them in the kitchen, where dinner preparations were under way.

"I can't. I can't move. Leave me alone."

They returned to the kitchen, and I started to cry. It was as if the tears were being drawn from my very marrow. I had my journal beside me, and I wrote:

All that fills my mind is the fact that Andrea has been condemned to live in her body. How can I find peace knowing she is alive? I see her little limbs trembling uncontrollably while her entire body labors to take a breath. I can't bear it.

In what seemed like the far distance, I could hear chairs scraping the floor and Lowell and Becky settling themselves at the table to eat. My concern not to upset my husband and my oldest buddy further finally prompted me to join them for dinner. I had been engulfed, buried alive with despondency, but I managed to come out of it.

Before Lowell went to work the next day, we made plans to rendezvous at the White Plains train station en route to my father's for an overnight stay. I then called West-One and spoke with a nurse by the name of Lillian, who reported that Andrea's IV had come out and had to be put back in. "She didn't spit up all night," she announced, as if this was good news. They had elevated her bed to help keep the formula (a mixture of cereal and Infamil) down.

I went to the pool, where I saw Leona; although we acknowledged each other, we did not speak. I imagined that she simply didn't know what to say. We had been pregnant at the same time and had fantasies of watching our babies play together. She must have felt that talking about her daughter would be too difficult for me. She must also have known that Dr. Stein had changed his mind and that Lowell and I were at odds with the hospital, her employer. From my point of view, on West-One she helped to keep babies alive, and some of them were babies who were trying to die, like Andrea. In light of all this, what could she say to me?

But when I got home from the club, there was a phone message from her. "At the pool, you seemed so upset. I just want you to know that I think of you and Lowell and Andrea."

While packing for my trip upstate, Bruce Maxwell phoned. I had called him earlier asking if he thought a legal battle to get Andrea's feedings stopped had any chance of success. Would he be willing to represent us?

"Feeding has never been withheld by a New York State

court, and New Jersey has only one case that I'm aware of. Not only would you never win, but you'd draw unpleasant attention to yourselves if the media got involved. You wouldn't want that." In an almost fatherly tone of voice he added, "You're just going to have to do some watchful waiting."

Then my Aunt Selma called. She had visited Andrea with my mother, so she had seen with her own eyes the tragedy of her condition. Selma was the only one of my extended family of aunts, uncles, and cousins who had had the courage to walk onto West-One. She was keeping herself informed of the latest developments, and she felt for us. My cousins and my sister, except for a few perfunctory phone calls early on, maintained their distance from me. If they wanted information, they'd call my mother.

"Selma, I have been considering killing Andrea myself," I said, sparing her nothing.

She gasped, then replied, "Deborah, you cannot do that. Lowell needs you, and ending up in jail would destroy your life and Lowell's. I don't want to hear you talk that way."

When we got off the phone I thought, "How could I expect her to understand? All I can do for Andrea as her mother, as her protector, is see to it that she doesn't remain trapped in that body. No one else will do that. I'm the only one."

My need to spare Andrea in this way was deep, primordial, and organic. I had the instincts of an animal who had to destroy her offspring because the young one was not equipped to survive on her own.

Along with my change of clothes and toiletries I packed my diaphragm. Lowell and I hadn't made love in three weeks, and I felt like I would never be able to experience pleasure again; but what the hell, I tossed it in my bag. Would Lowell still lust for me with a massive scar adorning my body, running across my belly like a crooked and rusty zipper? More important, could we let go of our grief long enough to connect sexually?

I went straight to the train station, braving a day without seeing Andrea. On board, sitting by a window, I watched neighborhoods of dilapidated streets and windowless buildings rush by, to be replaced by stretches of countryside and cozy towns encircling their train depots. I reflected on my doubts and fears about having another baby. I felt like our procreation was jinxed: first the miscarriage, then this. How could I take another chance? And if I ever was pregnant again, how could I give birth in a hospital?

I thought, "The hospital took Andrea away from me. The hospital took away my right, as her mother, to decide what should be done for her; and this happened the minute I checked in when I was in labor. This mess we are in, this horrible, horrible mess, is due to the inability of the doctors to do the humane thing for Andrea because some fucking lawyer who probably never saw Andrea in his life had to protect the hospital from . . . what? What are they afraid of?" Lawsuits? Criminal prosecution? Why couldn't they just put Andrea first?

At The Farm, my father, Kitty, Lowell, and I got together before dinner to strategize. My father, the consummate troubleshooter, saw the hospital's refusal to withhold nutrition as simply an obstacle to be overcome. We discussed the possibility of suing the hospital: whether we would win, what it would cost us emotionally and financially, and who would take such a case on. Kitty (a retired newspaper reporter) talked about leaking our story to the press in a way that would help our cause. But could we count on that? Then there was the possibility of finding a hospital somewhere in the world to which Andrea could be transferred that would honor our wishes.

Meanwhile, I was fighting to maintain an unruffled demeanor, to keep from spoiling our time with my parents with an emotional breakdown. When my voice would begin to waver or my eyes to swell with tears, my father would say, "Now Deb, try to keep cool." Much to my parents' disapproval, I expressed the need to call West-One, since I hadn't seen Andrea that day.

"Deborah, you have to start withdrawing from her and getting on with your life," my father counseled.

"Dad, it's only been twenty-three days since her birth."

Kitty interjected, "It's been longer than that if you consider the bonding you did with her when you were pregnant. It was as if you already had an Andrea in your life when she was in your womb."

I asked, "What do you mean?"

"Maybe it wasn't such a good idea after all to have learned of her sex and to have named her when she was in utero. You already had a relationship with her, and she wasn't even born yet. Maybe if that hadn't happened, your bond with her now wouldn't be so strong, and it wouldn't be as painful to let go."

I had never looked at it from that perspective. I felt I had to defend myself.

"Kitty, it wouldn't have made a difference if I'd never had a single sonogram or seen her image on a screen. I felt her inside of me. I carried her for nine months. She was part of me."

"Deb, you've got to start holding back or you'll lose yourself," my father said.

This led to a conversation about the beingness of Andrea. As Kitty put it, "Andrea doesn't exist. She's a beautiful baby doll, and the Andrea you wanted, who moved inside of you, is already dead."

Rationally, I knew she was right. They didn't want my life

to be ruined and my marriage to be threatened by my compulsion to assure Andrea's dying when in fact she was already dead in all but the most basic physical sense. But they were not yet sure whether to remove themselves from the situation or to fight, with Lowell and me, for Andrea's right to die. For them it was a matter of principle and moral obligation. They did not experience Andrea as a person, let alone a granddaughter.

My father and Kitty wanted me to "get on with my life" because they did not want to see me destroyed. But Andrea was not a corpse and she could not be buried and I could not abandon her. What they didn't understand was that dealing with Andrea *was* my way of getting on with my life. I was acting in the only way I could. I was in touch with my feelings, and I wasn't ready to relinquish my responsibility to her as her mother.

The next day, my parents came into the city with us. I called West-One the minute we all walked in the door of our apartment and learned that Andrea had been put in a crib. "A crib, like a real baby," I thought. I wanted to see her. It was a craving like an addiction.

My father and Lowell were discussing the medical records, which we had actually seen in a records office. "We went to the hospital to fill out yet another request for the records, and we walked into this office and saw our records laying right on top of a heap of papers on this woman's desk," Lowell explained.

"It could only mean they're preparing themselves," my father replied. "Where are the records now?"

"We're supposed to be getting them in the mail, minus the fetal monitor strips, which will be ready at a later date."

"Didn't Rick Pagan tell us that hospitals sometimes lose the strips or alter them?" I interjected.

Lowell said, "Oh yeah, he told us we shouldn't be surprised if we find that there are sheets missing from the strips."

The phone rang. It was someone from the English department at Pace University asking if I was still interested in an adjunct position, and if so, would I be able to come for an interview as soon as possible. It was like a call from another planet: this woman could have been a Martian asking me to teach on Mars. It had been a year since I mailed a resume and letters of recommendation to Pace. This was a most unexpected call. Revealing nothing of my current circumstances, I agreed to meet with the chairman of the department the next Monday. Somehow, some way, I would assume the character of a normal person of normal concerns and present myself as the English teacher and writer I once was, a long, long time ago.

When I got off the phone I said, "That was Pace University. I can't believe that I'm actually going to be interviewed Monday. I really don't know if I'll be able to pull it off."

"Sure you will," my father encouraged. I knew he was thinking that this was "getting on with my life."

My parents left for their studio, Lowell went to the health club, and I stayed home to make phone calls. I spoke first to David Schwartz, letting him know that we had decided to use his firm.

"I'd like to ask you one thing: what do we do with the hospital bills?" I asked.

"Submit them to your insurance company, do not pay any money out of your pocket, and keep a close record of correspondence with the insurance company," he instructed.

Already, by having a lawyer to turn to I felt I had a little control over what was happening to us.

I got in touch with the Society for the Right to Die, where a lawyer, Fenella Rouse, recommended that I speak with

Rose Gasner, also a lawyer there, whose area was infant cases. I stayed home awaiting a call from her.

The hours passed. Ms. Gasner did not get back to me, and I did not go to the hospital to see Andrea. I was suffering from withdrawal, but I knew if I saw her I would be devastated. I was beginning the process of letting go. I called, of course, and was told that she couldn't maintain her body temperature in the crib, so she was put back in the isolette.

I unpacked my bag, returned the untouched diaphragm to its drawer, and felt, for the first time, that Lowell and I would get back to each other, one of these days—when we were ready.

6

Despair

For Andrea

Even before I felt the kindling of life
flutter in my belly, I knew your presence
as a vision of cells separating into being.

I loved the thought of you: your beginning,
sacred genetic intermingling:
mommy's eyes and daddy's mouth,
generations of traits transformed in utero.

Then came subtle shoves of limbs
flexing through ribs,
occasional hiccups, then feet
protruding with fists through my skin.

You were a person to me.

My darling little girl,
I am dumb to explain your fate,
powerless to stop what you've become:
gone from your body
that breathes to feign life.

You are an innocent
with a soul like a halo
that encircles and waits
to merge with your body.

I so wanted you, baby,
to love and hold
feeding from my breasts.

Now all I want
is your corporeal death.

It was Father's Day, and the question was, do we acknowledge it? On Mother's Day I had been pregnant with Andrea; Lowell had gotten me a nightgown with buttons down the front for easy nursing. We had taken my mother out for a champagne brunch, and when we toasted to her I thought, "Next year, this will be my special day too."

Now Lowell was indeed a father, but we couldn't celebrate that fact. Instead we honored my father with a buffet brunch at a local restaurant. My father, knowing our financial state, contributed by buying a round of champagne. It was an occasion to get dressed up, to pretend, for the length of time it took to get through the meal, that our hearts weren't breaking, and to try to talk about things that had once amused us. My parents shared Lowell's enthusiasm for musical theater, and he shared theirs for opera, so our conversation focused on those sources of pleasure.

I had been thinking about writing a book, Andrea's story. My father and stepmother, who had coauthored several books, were always willing to discuss the conversion of experience into language. While there was an unspoken agreement not to talk about Andrea as she was at the moment—that would certainly have crashed our little party—it was permitted to talk about Andrea as the subject of a proposed book.

"Lowell might be able to borrow a computer from the high school during the summer. Of course, I'd have to learn how to use it," I said. I felt that I could somehow separate myself from the pain of the experience and have enough detachment to write about it.

My father and Kitty were encouraging. "This could be an important book in terms of family rights, the right to die, the abuses of medical technology, issues in neonatology. It would take at least a year of research," my father speculated.

"Our friend, Enez, sent me some journal articles on PVS, which stands for persistent vegetative state, a term I'd never heard of. There's so much to learn."

In fact, after reading these articles I had tried to get Dr. Hines to designate Andrea as being brain dead, comatose, or vegetative, because I thought such a distinction would make a difference regarding the withdrawal of nutrition. He was able to say she wasn't brain dead because the EEG wasn't completely flat, but whether she was in a coma, or in a PVS, he couldn't determine. He didn't elaborate, but I got the sense that the terms "coma" and "PVS" were inapplicable because of the newness of the brain, that an infant's brain waves were different from an adult's. It seemed that there just wasn't a term that described Andrea's condition. I thought that somehow it would make a difference if they could say she was in a coma or in a PVS, but I didn't know what difference. All I did know was that her brain was damaged so severely that her beingness, her personhood, was destroyed, but her body lived on. Dr. Hines did not explain further but simply sat, as usual, staring at me. I was feeling increasingly incensed and suspicious that he was withholding information.

That Father's Day afternoon, Lowell and I were feeling relaxed and intimate, and, with gentle consideration, we made love. It was soon apparent that we hadn't forgotten how, after the weeks of abstinence because of our emotional distress and my postpartum hormones. Being capable of giving and receiving pleasure in the midst of our despair seemed truly a gift. This connection made us more than the bereaved parents of Andrea: we were once again each other's mate. We passed the most normal day we had yet experienced since Andrea's birth, and I noted to myself that I hadn't cried once.

First thing Monday morning I called West-One and was told that Andrea was withdrawing from stimuli and had "cried out when tape was removed from her head." That she felt pain was something I had continually suspected and often agonized over. I thought, "My God, if she can feel the tape, what else must she feel? The needles, the tubes, the constant tugging at her body . . ." I couldn't think about it; it made me crazy. I called Dr. Maslin's office and left a message for her to call me. I hoped that, as Andrea's neurologist, she could tell me what Andrea might possibly feel.

My ability to accept that Andrea's destiny was out of my control fluctuated hour by hour. I could be swimming my laps at the pool, thrashing through the water, while wondering about the greater lesson I was supposed to learn. I'd consider that Andrea was mine to the extent that any person belongs to someone else—which is, not at all. She was her own person, and I was the vessel through which she had passed.

This perspective would relieve me momentarily, as I burdened mother nature with the responsibility of assuring what was best for my baby. I'd get out of the pool with this enlightened outlook. It would last thirty minutes at the most, only to dissipate into the rationalization that it really was. In the end, no thought, idea, or mental leap could annihilate the anguish that gripped me.

Before I left for my interview at Pace University, Rose Gasner, from the Society for the Right to Die, finally returned my call. Our conversation revolved around the term "appropriate," as in "appropriate nutrition." The issue was not merely one of semantics, though my increasing cynicism tended to treat it as such. Unbelievably, Andrea's fate rested on how this word was interpreted.

The hospital, it seemed, was legally obligated to give appropriate care, a concept that has always included nutrition and hydration. Providing food and water for all patients, no matter how severe their condition, was considered basic and humane. Furthermore, doctors who did not provide appropriate care for newborns could be found guilty of child abuse and neglect; if death was the result, they could also be found guilty of manslaughter.

Yet for Andrea, who could not suck and who would never be capable of self-feeding (like the many adults in persistent vegetative states who are fed through tubes, artificially), were nutrition and hydration appropriate, or were they just another form of life support that was intrusive and defied the integrity of the individual? If Andrea was perceived as already dying, not as living, her death by starvation would be a natural end to her existence. In that case, any doctors who aided in her death would not be guilty of manslaughter; they would simply have allowed nature to take its course.

I had to draw upon my college philosophy courses to analyze what we were up against, recalling distinctions in logic and ethics that had once been purely intellectual challenges to articulate in class. Little did I know, when I was a student assisting a professor of ethics by compiling lists of references to euthanasia, that I would one day be caught in the unresolved issues of what indeed constituted passive euthanasia (the withdrawing of nutrition and hydration) and what constituted murder. This question was now far from academic.

Then Rose Gasner and I discussed the Cruzan case, which Kathy Nolan had mentioned. Nancy Cruzan, at the age of twenty-five, had been in a car accident that left her deprived of oxygen for at least fourteen minutes. Upon the arrival of the ambulance, paramedics resuscitated her. Only her brain stem was intact, but she was able to breathe on her own. Her parents, incapable of projecting into the future of her rehabilitation, consented to the insertion of a feeding tube directly into her stomach, a procedure known as a gastrostomy. Six years later, Nancy remained in a persistent vegetative state; her parents sought a court order to have the feeding tube removed, since clearly she would never recover. Their local probate court granted the necessary permission, but the assistant attorney general for the state of Missouri appealed to the Missouri Supreme Court, which ruled against the Cruzans on the grounds that life must at all costs be preserved. In the opinion of the court, there was insufficient evidence that Nancy herself would have requested the removal of the feeding tube. Furthermore, the court ruled, the Cruzans did not have the right, as legal guardians, to make that decision for their daughter.

This ruling did not bode well for our situation. Complicating matters was the fact that in our case it was impossible to know what Andrea herself might have wanted—whether to continue to live given her condition, or to be allowed to die.

The Cruzans were going to appeal their case to the U.S. Supreme Court, and it was the outcome of this appeal that we had to await.

"Ms. Gasner, it seems to me that there is not one human being in the entire universe who would want to remain in

Nancy Cruzan's state. Even a mentally retarded person could see that this is not a life. It is beyond belief that the parents have to endure further heartache to prove this. I really think the issue is not about protecting life, but about denying our mortality. Don't you agree? Medical technology makes death something that is not natural and that should be avoided by all possible means. What else could explain what is happening in Missouri?''

"I agree that this is part of it," she said. She also agreed that it was inappropriate to feed Andrea, given her condition and prognosis, but she concluded: "I don't think our involvement will help you—that is to say, involvement from the outside." She said she would like to speak with Dr. Alan Fleischman, a neonatologist and ethicist at the Albert Einstein College of Medicine (whose reputation was on a par with Dr. Cassell's), regarding the word "appropriate." I encouraged her to do so. Despite the inability of her organization to help directly, I was glad to have found someone else who not only understood our position but supported it as well.

The more I spoke with people whose professional work touched on aspects of Andrea's situation, the more aware I became that what applied to incompetent adults, in terms of medical treatment and legal implications, did not necessarily apply to newborns. With newborns there was an element of the unknown, of their unpredictable power of self-healing and resiliency. It was harder to deem a newborn beyond hope; consequently, it was harder to turn off life support. Babies, after all, were the pinnacle of life, brimming with human potential. We were traveling in uncharted terrain.

At Pace University, I sat before the chairman of the English department and the second in command, wearing the same brown dress I had worn for all the recent occasions that had required me to put on my public persona. I felt like an impostor. Dr. Raskin, the chairman, was courteous and either didn't notice or didn't let on that he noticed that I was distracted and a touch possessed. They knew that I had been running a reading series for writers of poetry and prose, some of whom taught in the department, and we talked about that. My past experience teaching emotionally disturbed teenagers was also an advantage, for they wanted me to teach basic writing and literature to freshman students who, because of behavioral problems that had acted as academic barriers in high school, were not yet ready for the standard Pace curriculum. The longer we talked, the easier it became to summon my past life and find the words that corresponded to what we were discussing. I felt professionally confident that I could handle the courses and the students.

When it came time to explain what I had been up to in the recent past, I had no choice but to tell them that I had been pregnant, had given birth, and was in the midst of a nightmarish ordeal. I was reticent about sharing too much, but their empathy allowed me to be honest about the circumstances. We parted with their good wishes and a request that I return to meet the dean of arts and sciences.

I walked off the Pace campus feeling proud that I had convinced them and myself that I was who I was, who my resume said I was. The real test would be whether I could suspend my preoccupation with Andrea enough to expound on commas, semicolons, and sentence fragments as well as on the beauty of language, which I once held so dear.

I called West-One upon my return and learned that because of monthly rotations Dr. Stein had been replaced by a Dr. Kravitz. This was the man my father's contact at the hospital knew. Although it was our understanding that Dr. Kravitz might be more receptive to our wishes for Andrea, I could not let myself get optimistic. Dr. Maslin never got back to me. Indeed, I was finding that as the days and weeks wore on, none of Andrea's various doctors were returning my calls.

After dinner I went straight to bed and wept. I said to Lowell, who lay beside me, "All I can think about is her crying out in pain when that tape was peeled off her head. She must feel everything, every prick with a needle, every nudge of the tube down her nose and throat—everything. And I don't understand why that fucking doctor couldn't call me back. It's so goddamn frustrating."

"Deb, honey, she probably didn't get the message. She may work at other hospitals too."

Then the real source of my anguish surfaced, what lay beneath my consciousness. I thought, "If she feels pain, she could feel comfort, she could feel caresses." My sobbing increased. It had been five days since I had last seen her, since I had held her, touched her. I felt guilty and confused. I couldn't even talk about it.

Lowell, holding me, repeated, "Let it go, let it go." He added, "Deb, you mustn't lose faith in us."

The next morning, I called Dr. Kravitz to set up an appointment. I reiterated our desire that Andrea's feedings be stopped. While he sympathized with us, he said, "It's against the law to starve a baby. She will be receiving custodial care." He didn't sound much different from Dr. Stein. Then he informed me that she had been moved to a special nursery where they kept "healthier babies," because West-One had run out of room. He also mentioned that her feedings had increased.

I thought, "Great, now when we visit her we can see all the healthier babies." Aloud I said simply, "Okay, Dr. Kravitz, see you tomorrow morning." As I signed off, I felt a wave of despair come over me.

It was Lowell's day off from the high school, and he was home with several voice lessons lined up. We decided that I would go alone to meet with our lawyer, Ricky Pagan, for we had finally secured the records.

I found Ricky in his office, colossal stacks of paper covering every inch of his desk. The surrounding carpet was also concealed beneath documents heaped in precarious piles that seemed on the verge of toppling over. As he reached over this immense disarray to shake hands I thought, "It must be hell being a lawyer."

"Have a seat. Would you like some coffee?"

"No thank you. Here are the records," I said, handing over my precious bundle.

I sat in silence, watching him carefully as he leafed through the hospital's account of my labor and Andrea's birth.

At long last he spoke. "You know, it's not often that you have everything right in front of you. I mean, everything's here, except the strips, which, unless there are pages missing, will correspond with this report."

"What do you find? What do you see?" I was on the edge of my seat. At last I would hear a hypothesis to explain what went wrong.

"Look, let me try to get Dr. Berman on the phone. He's one of our expert witnesses."

"Which means?"

"We have doctors, experts in their fields, who review the records and evaluate the possibility of negligence. Usually, if I don't have everything laid out in front of me, I mail the records and wait for a report. But let me see if I can reach him. Let's see if he can tell me anything over the phone."

"What do you suspect?" I asked as he prepared to make the call.

"I think the Pitocin which was given to you unsupervised and without proper monitoring. My guess is, that's what caused the fetal distress."

"What do you mean, 'without proper monitoring'? The midwife told me she was giving it to me."

"Yes. But as far as you remember, you weren't examined by an obstetrician beforehand. Am I correct?"

"Yes."

"Well, I think that's a requirement."

"Wow" was all I could say.

While Ricky spoke with Dr. Berman I sat in the chair and relived that portentous moment when June announced that she would be inducing my labor with Pitocin and how my gut reaction had been to reject it. I thought, "He's right. Ricky is right. It had to have been the Pitocin. Oh God, if only I had followed my instinct."

I was half listening to his conversation as I concentrated on keeping my emotions in check and my eyes from over-flowing. All I could think was, "I could have prevented it. I should have been more assertive. I should have insisted." I was enmeshed in this self-flagellation when Ricky got off the phone, breaking my spell.

"Well, Dr. Berman concurs. Of course, he needs to see the records firsthand, but on the basis of what I told him, a synopsis, he thinks you probably should not have been given Pitocin at all, but in any case you should have been examined by the obstetrician first."

"Why shouldn't I have been given any?"

"Because you were in labor. You were having contractions. Pitocin is usually given to induce labor, to get the contractions going. For some reason the baby wasn't descending, and the Pitocin may have made matters worse. It could have intensified the contractions and cut off the baby's oxygen."

"Oh."

"When do you think you'll have the strips?"

I searched for my voice. "Hopefully by the end of the week. I have to pick them up."

"Look, I'm terribly sorry. I know this is tragic for you and your husband, and I hope things work out the way you want them. From my end I can say I think there is negligence here, and we will pursue the case."

"Thank you. I'll try to get the strips to you on Friday, as soon as I pick them up." We shook hands.

I had been with Ricky for nearly three hours; I felt drained. In that state of unreality that was becoming all too familiar, I made my way underground, through subway stations, trains, and tunnels, back to our apartment.

Lowell was just finishing a voice lesson when I got home. I sat on the couch waiting for him, ruminating over my time with Ricky. We had also discussed getting court consent to stop Andrea's feedings. He felt that would be nearly impossible. He had found out that New York State had the toughest laws in the country regarding the withdrawal of life support, and besides, artificial feeding wasn't considered life support. I had said, "I didn't realize that each state had different policies. Maybe there's a state we can transfer her to that's more lenient."

"You'd still have to get her released," he reminded me.

Charlie, Lowell's student, emerged from the music room and expressed his sorrow for our situation. After he had gone Lowell and I lay down on the bed—as had by now become our custom when discussing news of Andrea—to talk about my meeting with Ricky.

"He thinks we definitely have a case. He thinks, along with the doctor, the expert witness, that it was the injudicious use of Pitocin that caused fetal distress. I probably shouldn't have been given any, and I certainly should have been examined beforehand and monitored by Dr. Kembel. I never saw Kembel until the end, until the C-section. But apparently he signed for the Pitocin."

Lowell let out a sigh. We held each other. I said, "I feel responsible. I know it's irrational. . . . I know it was June's decision and that I had no choice but to trust her. But still . . . Do you remember how I immediately said I didn't want any?"

"Honey, you can't blame yourself. If anyone was responsible, I think it was June and Kembel. You were in no shape to make any kind of decision. None of us was. They were in charge. Please, please don't blame yourself."

That evening we spoke with a nurse who reported that Andrea was getting some of my thawed breast milk with rice cereal mixed in, and that the IV had been removed because she was tolerating the feedings; however, she still needed suctioning every three hours.

I fell asleep with the vision of Andrea in the special nursery, with plump babies gurgling around her as she imperceptibly grew longer and fatter. They were doing what they said they'd do: they were keeping her alive.

We decided to see Andrea after, rather than before, our morning meeting with Dr. Kravitz. In his office we were joined by Gloria and Enid; we hadn't seen or spoken to either of them in days. Gloria was receptive and concerned, but Enid appeared defensive and cautious. Dr. Kravitz was light years away from Stein in terms of social skills and warmth. It was apparent that he was a man of compassion; nevertheless, his hands were tied. He was not a maverick, and he wouldn't rock the boat. As they saw things, the point of the meeting was to discuss placement for Andrea upon her release—and they weren't talking about another hospital that would let her die, either. I simply could not project into a future that included Andrea. I had been in institutions for the incurable; I would not envision for even a second Andrea's presence in such a place.

"Dr. Kravitz, there is no point to this. Why assure her such a life, to rot in a bed in some miserable warehouse. I haven't got what it takes to think about placements. Besides, she's your baby anyway. You'll have to deal with her."

"Excuse me?" he responded.

"You won't release her into our care and you won't transfer her to a hospital that might do what we want, what is best for her. So, she's yours. You find a placement for her."

"Mrs. Alecson, please understand, for us to do that will require legal action on your part to relinquish custody."

I interrupted, "But I don't have custody. If I did, she wouldn't be here."

I couldn't help myself. Although I could hear Dr. Cassell's voice in the back of my mind advising me to maintain good relations with the hospital, to avoid, at all costs, an adversarial situation, I couldn't stop. I was out of control. I would not cooperate.

Lowell silenced me with his eyes and talked reasonably about the legal procedure to surrender custody. "Are there institutions for her? Can you really place her? Is there someone we need to talk to?" he asked.

I glared at him, for he was siding with the enemy, making it too easy for them.

From this point on, Dr. Kravitz directed his conversation to Lowell, while I sat in a constrained huff thinking, "It doesn't matter what I say, what we want. They'll do what they have to do."

Lowell got the name of the woman whose task it was to find placements. He told Dr. Kravitz that we'd make an appointment as I walked out of the office without shaking the doctor's hand. Gloria led us to Andrea's nursery and informed us that she was no longer her primary nurse because of the transfer, a fact that only added to my feelings of anger and impotence. Before, at least we had had Gloria.

There she lay in an isolette, looking a little more bloated and distorted than when last we had seen her. With eyes closed and her body limp, she seemed inanimate. Lowell and I stood side by side peering down at her. "She looks retarded, you know what I mean, she has that look that some retarded people have," I said. Lowell shook his head. After several minutes of gazing upon her, we turned to leave. Lowell walked ahead of me, and I surveyed the room, then quickly unplugged what I assumed to be the thermostat on her isolette. It was an unpremeditated move, a desperate gesture. No bells went off, no signals flashed. I scurried out of the nursery like a criminal.

Before leaving the hospital, Lowell picked up Andrea's bill, out of curiosity. It came to $31,000. We looked it over during the bus ride home and concluded that it might just as well have been $31,000,000 given our financial situation. It was so outrageous that we couldn't take it seriously.

At home again, I spoke with Ben, who called wanting to know if we had met with Bruce Maxwell, his recommendation for a possible attorney. I described what had transpired between us and said that we had decided on a different firm. I also gave him a mini report on Andrea's status. Before we hung up he said, "If there's anything I can do, please don't hesitate to ask."

"Well, actually, there is something you can do. You can get me some poison."

There was silence on the other end.

"What?"

"Poison."

"You're kidding, aren't you?"

"No."

"Well, I'll see what I can do." I knew that I had crossed a line with him, but I was serious.

Then my father called wanting to know of new developments. I told him about our meeting with Dr. Kravitz. "Dr. Kravitz, deep down, agrees with us about letting her die. He talked about his mother, who had Alzheimer's and lingered for years while he and his brother tried to get life support withdrawn. There they were, two doctors, and they couldn't do anything. So he understands. He said something about if Andrea was in a small hospital in some obscure town somewhere, she probably would never have reached this point. His hospital is often in the limelight, and they can't risk drawing attention to themselves."

"Well, if you could have her transferred to the local hospital up here, she'd be sure to die. You put your life on the line when you enter that place."

I laughed. My father always had the knack for seeing the absurdity in things and for relieving other people's stress with his jokes.

It was time to make dinner. The only thing I had enough imagination to think of was scrambled eggs, baked potatoes, and a steamed vegetable, but I hadn't the wherewithal to accomplish even that. Lowell assembled our meal, and I mechanically ate what was on the plate. Afterward, I retreated to our bed, where I sat and stared into the darkness. I thought about killing Andrea and about Lowell's nearing departure for Minnesota. That would be an opportune time to do it.

Within twenty-four hours, Lowell was to leave for his nephew's wedding in Minnesota. The family had asked that he sing for the occasion. They'd invited me too, but I couldn't bring myself to attend a happy gathering with people I did not know well. I turned on a light and wrote in my journal:

> I wish Lowell wasn't going, but I'd never ask him to stay home. He wants to go and it will probably be good for him. I can't face a bunch of people I don't know for a celebratory gathering. And the traveling itself seems more than I can physically bear.
>
> Oh God—how do I get on with my life?
>
> Today I am dulled & sad & disappointed. And I'm afraid.
> I'm afraid to be without Lowell even for three nights
> and I'm afraid to carry another child
> and I'm afraid I won't experience joy again
> and I'm afraid Andrea will live on and on
> and I'm afraid that my suffering will never end.

The few words I exchanged with Lowell after dinner had to do with his trip. I told him, "I wish you weren't going." To which he replied, "What will that do?" I knew I was being unfair and that I was provoking an argument, but I couldn't help it. I got myself worked up and stormed out the door with this sense that I just had to escape the apartment. Retrieving my bag and journal, I stepped onto the streets of Manhattan, destination unknown.

I wound up in a restaurant several blocks from home. I sat at a table near the window, ordered a glass of wine, and began to write disjointedly:

> I can't stab her. I haven't the guts. I think of ways: choking, suffocating, throwing her across the room—but there will be people around. So I think—how can I abduct her? Should I try tomorrow night/morning, like 2 A.M. when Lowell's in Minnesota? How will I do it? Take a cab and have it wait? I'll need help. I'll need someone

to hold the elevator while I grab Andrea, unhook her, and evade the nurses.

I am regressing.

The nursery is as it was—prepared for Andrea. Her toys are out. I carried a perfect baby.

Lowell was waiting for me when I returned. He had been packing for the trip, but when I came in he embraced me.

That night I dreamt that I was on the subway and sitting across from me was a toddler. She stared at me with wide eyes, and I realized that she was Andrea. She was with a woman—her adopted mother, I assumed. She looked hurt. I felt that I had abandoned her.

The next morning I woke up to find a new face lying beside mine. It took several seconds to realize what the difference was. "Ah, you've shaved your mustache! You look adorable. What made you do that?"

"I felt it was time for a change," Lowell answered, smiling.

After breakfast he left for the airport, and I went to pick up the fetal monitor strips. I had to go to a building on the Upper West Side, almost in Harlem. I found the room where I was to rendezvous with someone, I assumed, from the hospital. I knocked on the door; no one answered. I began to feel paranoid, as if this was a setup. Those strips might help to prove negligence by the hospital, along with June and Kembel. I waited around a poorly lit hall for what felt like hours before a man approached and, without addressing me, unlocked the door. I followed him inside, making sure to keep the door from slamming shut. I told him I was there for the strips. He apparently expected this, and he gave me a packet. Before leaving I said, "Are you sure they're all here?" He answered sharply, "I'm sure."

Traveling all the way downtown to Ricky's office, I found that I was a bit shaken. It was as if I had just completed a dangerous mission of espionage, and in my possession were highly charged and confidential documents.

I delivered the strips into Ricky's hands and sat silently while he looked through them. I had tried to decipher the graph myself, but I couldn't interpret the ups and downs. Ricky was amazed to find that all the pages were present. In his opinion they indicated fetal distress, in the form of decelerations. He pointed these out to me; they appeared as major plunges in an otherwise steady horizontal line.

"These may be what Dr. Kembel saw and discussed with June," I said. I was remembering the incident before it was decided I'd need a Caesarean.

"Well, everything's here now. I'll send them off to Dr. Berman," he said as we parted.

I had planned to spend the weekend, while Lowell was away, with my father and stepmother at The Farm. Before leaving to catch my train upstate I picked up a book I had ordered on Kathy Nolan's recommendation, *Playing God in the Nursery* by Jeff Lyon, a reporter for the *Chicago Tribune*. The book, Kathy said, was about neonatal intensive care units and the medical, legal, and ethical issues involved in crisis care of infants. It sounded like the perfect book for me.

I made myself comfortable on the Brewster-bound train, my feet propped up on the seat across from mine, and started on Lyon's book. The first chapter was called "Baby Doe," and this is what I learned:

On April 9, 1982, following a normal and full-term pregnancy, a baby boy was born to a woman in Bloomington, Indiana, who became known as Mrs. Doe. It was immediately evident to the obstetrician, Dr. Owens, that the baby had Down's syndrome; but that was the least of his problems. Meconium was found in the amniotic fluid (this often indicates fetal distress). The newborn had a disastrous Apgar score of two and was blue in appearance owing to oxygen deprivation. The baby had an esophageal atresia (an abnormal esophagus) and a suspected tracheo-esophageal fistula (in which the esophagus enters the windpipe directly, making breathing and the clearing of mucus difficult).

Dr. Owens, wanting a second opinion, called upon Dr. Schaffer, a pediatrician used by the Doe family. Schaffer found all the malformations that Dr. Owens had found, as well as an enlarged heart as seen on the chest X-ray.

Finally, the Does' general practitioner, Dr. Wenzler, was summoned, and the three physicians conferred. All agreed on the condition of the child, and they presented their findings to the Does soon after the birth. With the exception of the Down's syndrome, the birth defects were treatable. Dr. Schaffer advised that the baby be transferred to another facility, Riley Children's Hospital, where surgery could be performed. Without the operation, the baby would die. Dr. Wenzler supported that assessment. It was Dr. Owens who changed the course of neonatal history when he disagreed, recommending instead that the Does do nothing and let the child die. He told the parents that the surgical procedure was painful, that followup surgery would be necessary, and that the child's mental retardation from Down's syndrome could be severe.

The Does took time to discuss the situation in private with their closest friends, who were present at the hospital. After thirty minutes or so they reached a decision: not to treat the baby.

Up until this point, everything made sense. The Does received three expert opinions and then carefully weighed their options. They were both teachers—as Lowell and I were—and the father, who had worked with handicapped children—as I had—felt that Down's children rarely had good lives. Furthermore, they had two other children to consider. They didn't want to burden their family with the care of what would certainly be a profoundly compromised individual who would need constant medical attention. In a sane and compassionate world, the Does would have kept a vigil by their son's side, had him baptized perhaps (as they did, for they were Catholic), and prepared for his death. Their decision would have been respected by the medical personnel at the hospital, and they would have been given the space and grace to accept their disappointment and mourn their loss. The boy would have died, being spared a horrific existence, he would have been buried or cremated, and the Does would have gone on with their lives.

But Dr. Schaffer could not leave well enough alone, for in his mind what they were proposing was infanticide. He called the head of the NICU at Riley and told him what was happening. He threatened Dr. Owens with legal action. By now, the hospital administrators were becoming worried as well: they didn't want to be held liable. They wanted the Does, against their wishes, to take the child home rather than leave him to die in their hospital.

The hospital's lawyer came up with a solution: he requested a judicial hearing with the hope that the judge would either order that the child be sent to Riley or remove custody from the parents.

A hearing was convened, attended by the father and the lawyers, doctors, and hospital administrators. After hearing from everyone, Judge Baker ruled that the Does had every right to choose one of the two treatment plans proposed; this they had done, and therefore the baby should be permitted to die.

However, the story did not end there. In the name of preserving life, complete strangers to the Does made further appeals, and the couple had to endure more meetings and more directives until the child died, six days after his birth. Even then they weren't free from harassment inflicted by right-to-life advocates.

Doctors, nurses, hospital administrators, lawyers, judges, attorney generals, right-to-life proponents, prospective adoptive parents, newspaper reporters, neighbors of the Does, government officials, and ultimately the president of the United States, Ronald Reagan, became involved, making what should have been one family's private grief an issue of political and ethical import. I had just started the section about the Reagan administration's actions and its development of the so-called Baby Doe regulations when the train pulled into Brewster North.

My father was waiting for me at the station. During the brief ride to The Farm I told him about what I had been reading. As we pulled into the driveway, I had a flashback to the time Lowell and I had found that baby doe resting on the gravel against the picket fence. Baby Doe. It was a message from Andrea.

7

Separation

On Saturday morning my father and I went grocery shopping at the local supermarket, where the aisles and checkout lines were filled with children of all shapes and sizes: babies hanging from mothers in Snugglies, toddlers strapped into the shopping cart seats, and assorted little ones demanding this or that from the plethora of items on the shelves. There were more children than adults in the store, few men, and it seemed that all the women either had offspring in tow or else were pregnant. Not knowing if my perception was skewed, I commented to my father, "Have you noticed that all the women in here are either mothers or about to be, and everyone, including the children, is overweight?"

"What else is there to do in Putnam County except eat and fuck?" my father joked.

We were searching the cans of coffee for a specific brand when I started to cry. I trailed behind my father, biting my lower lip in an attempt to stop the deluge. My father, soon aware of my agitation, softly said, "Deb, you'll have your baby one day." I turned away to find myself facing boxes of breakfast cereals. Through tears, confronted by a bowl of bran flakes and smiling raisins in milk, I thought, "It's impossible."

Back at The Farm, Kitty told us that Dr. Cassell had called and she had spoken with him. Of their conversation she said, "He told me that you should have never been allowed to hold Andrea and to bond with her."

"It's too late now. Besides, I don't know if it would have made any difference," I said.

Earlier that week, Dr. Cassell had made a statement that I found enigmatic. I was ranting and raving about how I had to set Andrea's soul free: "She is trapped in that body and I have to free her soul."

He replied, "You make a soul; you're not born with one."

I thought, "This is coming from a famous ethicist," and I asked him: "You make your soul?"

"Yes, a soul is not something you're born with; it is something you create."

"How does he know?" I wondered. "Could he be right?"

It was the kind of idea I thrived on, something I could mull over.

This question of how much I was willing to sacrifice for Andrea—or, in my parents' minds, this problem of my attachment to her—was one we touched on throughout my visit. When I mentioned my fantasies of killing her myself, my father didn't accept that her brief presence in my life could warrant such an extreme act. He said, "It would be another story if Andrea was in our lives for a number of years and had become a member of our family." That, to me, was like saying that a woman who had a miscarriage in the first trimester shouldn't feel devastated because she could have gone the whole nine months and had a stillbirth.

Meanwhile, my mother was continuing to see Andrea at

least once a week. This, I knew, my father and Kitty found to be excessive, perhaps even a little deranged. They had seen Andrea twice: when she was born and in that one visit to the NICU early on. They were trying to protect themselves. What was the point of making trips to look at an infant who would never be a real grandchild? As far as they were concerned, seeing her wouldn't change things, but it would make them depressed.

With my parents, I felt the need to defend my feelings regarding Andrea. They applauded me on my current suspension of visits, but in their eyes my calls to the NICU still needed to be decreased, if not eliminated.

When I had last spoken with a nurse on West-One, the evening I arrived at The Farm, she reported that Andrea was comfortable.

I asked, "How do you know?"

"Because I'm a mother," she replied.

This kind of interchange only tormented me further. It was no surprise that my parents wished I'd spare myself.

That evening in bed I read about the Baby Doe regulations. They were formulated in 1983 under the auspices of Dr. C. Everett Koop, the Reagan-appointed surgeon general, and released by the Department of Health and Human Services (HHS) to appease the right-to-life movement and various disability groups who were responding to the handling of Baby Doe and of another baby born soon after, in Illinois, whose parents refused permission for surgery to treat myelomeningocele (the worst form of spina bifida). Issued in conjunction with the regulations, which targeted hospitals and institutions that received federal funds, was a poster that was to be displayed on maternity floors and in nurseries. It read, "Discriminatory failure to feed and care for handicapped infants in this facility is prohibited by federal law," and encouraged anyone aware of infants being denied food or customary care to call a "Handicapped Infant Hotline," which was in service around the clock. This "anyone" need not have any connection with the infant. Complaints, if they sounded legitimate, were examined by a "Baby Doe squad," a team of investigators from state and federal governments. An inquiry would ensue, involving a thorough going-over of the baby's records and time-consuming interviews with the medical personnel involved. If discrimination was found to have occurred, the hospital in question could lose federal funding and the doctors could be found guilty of child abuse and neglect.

The most obvious flaw in the regulations was the labeling of all physical and mental defects merely as handicaps, not taking into account the severity or irreversibility of some conditions. In other words, the regulations mandated medically aggressive treatment of every baby, no matter what the affliction.

Before dozing off, I remembered Gloria once mentioning a poster hanging in the NICU not too long before. Judging by the way everyone was dealing with Andrea, I thought, the poster, if not actually there in black and white, certainly existed as a phantom in people's memories.

The next morning, Sunday, Lowell and I spoke on the telephone. He was feeling sad because there were a lot of children at the wedding. I would be leaving my father's at about the same time he'd be leaving Minnesota. We would converge at our apartment for a late dinner.

Riding home on the train, I considered what it would be like to place Andrea in an institution and whether we could or would disown her, if that act was necessary for us to get on with our lives. It was the first time I had projected into a future that included her existence somewhere in the world, but apart from me. My parents were undoubtedly having an influence. Then too, as brief as my visit was, any time out of the city seemed to give me enough emotional distance to reflect on Andrea and my obligation to her in a new light. Whether or not this detachment would last was another story.

The moment I walked into the apartment, I called West-One. I was told that Andrea's eyes were open. "It could be reflex," the nurse said.

I was sitting on the couch, summoning the vision of her as a porcelain doll with glass eyes, when Lowell got home. As he unpacked he talked about the wedding, the songs he sang for the ceremony and the reception, and about being with his family. "I saw my cousin Paul and his wife, Jane, and their two daughters for the first time in about eight or nine years. We were standing around having fruit punch, before the buffet, and they asked me how things were. They said, 'You must be going through a terrible time,' or something like that, and I started to answer, but I burst into tears."

"Then what happened?"

"I pulled myself together. You know, there were at least a hundred and fifty people socializing in this fellowship hall. I told them, 'Yes, it has been a nightmare,' but I couldn't really go into any details. It was a relief to talk a little about it, though, and to have them acknowledge what I was going through. Many of my other relatives said nothing, for fear, I guess, of upsetting me."

Indeed, we were finding that the world was divided between those who could talk to us and those who could not. Many people, I assumed, wouldn't mention Andrea because they thought it might bring our sorrow to the surface and cause us greater grief. Didn't they realize that she was on our minds regardless, every minute of every hour, awake or asleep? People didn't know what to say, and the simple words "I'm sorry this has happened to you" were often out of reach, too difficult to express.

The week began with Lowell taking a four-day computer course at the high school and with my meeting the dean at Pace. The meeting was a formality, for it was already decided that I would have the position. Somehow we got on the topic of the Hastings Center, and he told me that the center was housed on the Pace campus in Westchester—a fortuitous coincidence, I thought. I was welcomed aboard, introduced to whoever was around in the English department, and given a set of keys. I felt the thrill and terror of having obligated myself to teaching responsibilities that would require a clarity of thought I was far from certain I would possess come September.

Later that afternoon, I made a few phone calls. I had purchased a book called *The Right to Die*, by Derek Humphry and Ann Wickett. The authors were cofounders of the Hemlock Society in Los Angeles; I called their organization and left a message for Humphry on an answering machine. I thought maybe he'd have some ideas.

I then got in touch with the National Hospice Organization and learned that hospice services are more often than not given at home, or provided in settings that cater to short-term care. The hospital wouldn't release Andrea into our custody, so we couldn't take her home; and a hospice facility couldn't provide for her potentially long-term needs.

I phoned Ricky Pagan and asked him if we could legally disown Andrea.

"I never heard of such a thing," he replied. "What for? You can always walk away." Then he added, "But you're not ready to."

By the end of the day, after having heard again and again that there was nothing to be done for Andrea except to leave her at the mercy of the NICU administrators, I felt discouraged and numb. I could not, as Ricky suggested, "walk away," and neither could Lowell; but he was better able than I to focus on matters unrelated to Andrea.

I was beginning to experience the slightest rift between us as we coped in our separate ways. When I wasn't spending my time at Andrea's side, I was fully occupied by efforts to attain what we thought was best for her. Lowell, for his part, went to the high school, worked with voice students, and carried on as a professional person in the world. My existence was undefined: a woman who had given birth but wasn't a mother.

I went for a swim early the next morning. In the pool, I pondered the feasibility of bringing our case before a judge. What if the media learned of our situation? Would a headline appear in the local newspaper: "Couple Begs Judge to Starve Their Baby to Death"? Would we then be preyed upon by throngs of zealots marching outside our apartment building chanting, "Death to the child murderers"? What would it cost to hire a lawyer, and how could we even afford one? If we lost, what then?

One minute, it seemed, I could give myself the latitude to contemplate disowning her if she was to end up in some institution, while the next minute I was convinced, in the depths of my soul, that I could not live if that was to be her fate and that I had to prevent such an outcome: it was imperative.

Before leaving for a therapy session with Dr. Melner that afternoon, I contacted the New York State Task Force on Life and the Law and spoke with someone who expressed sympathy: "It is very difficult for parents at this time, there are no legal provisions, and infants cannot have proxies." This brought to mind a comment Kathy Nolan had made about our being "in a bad place in history." There was no judicial precedent in our favor, which made the Cruzan case in Missouri all the more crucial.

In despair, I called Kathy Nolan; my calls to her were becoming a daily routine. Of everyone I knew and spoke with, family and friends and all the doctors and nurses, I felt that she best understood not only the legal, moral, and medical implications of our situation but also the complexity of my pain. She was like a therapist, best friend, and authority all rolled into one. It was as if she had experienced the exact same thing at some time in her life—that's how deep her empathy was.

"Kathy, I am actually thinking about what to do, where to send Andrea, when the hospital is ready to discharge her. This is a big step for me, considering that up until this point all I could think about was how to kill her. I'm trying to find out if there's a place somewhere on earth that will eventually let her die."

Kathy's concern was with how I expressed to others what I wanted for Andrea. She knew what I meant when I said I wanted Andrea to die, but others might misconstrue. "When talking to people about Andrea," she advised, "don't say, 'We want the baby to die'; say, 'We know that the baby is dying and we don't want medical intervention.'"

No matter how I worded it, though, to ask that they—the institutions, the government, the lawyers for the hospitals—respect Andrea's right to die by not force-feeding her was to ask the unthinkable.

"Kathy, I also continue to think about fighting the hospital, bringing this to court, challenging the Baby Doe regulations. I go from pillar to post."

"Of course bringing her home would be the best thing. Infants and feeding tubes are a bad combination in New York. I don't know if yours would be a good test case. But if you should decide to seek legal action, I can help you get a lawyer."

Getting back to our discussion of placements, Kathy wondered if perhaps the original pediatrician I had chosen for her, Dr. Minsky, might be able to suggest something. Then she introduced the strong possibility that Andrea would develop an infection, pneumonia for instance, and that we might request that she not be given antibiotics.

"You can ask Dr. Kravitz how they would treat her if she had an infection."

I had never thought of this. I felt like I had been hit by a bolt of lightning. Of course—a way out: an infection. Kathy explained that because of her immobility and the buildup of fluids in her lungs, she would most likely have respiratory problems.

"Come to think of it," I said, "it seems that she needs more suctioning all the time. What if they suctioned her less? Would that promote infection?" I was virtually plotting Andrea's death. "And what about the seizures—the phenobarbital: if she didn't get that, could she die of continually having seizures?"

"Seizures may or may not interrupt breathing. A baby can seize for months. Withholding suctioning seems reasonable. Maybe there's a placement for her where the doctors won't order a feeding tube or an IV."

"If she didn't have the IV and had only oral feedings, then there'd be more secretions, which means more buildup, which means more risk of infections."

"Yes."

"But there's still the issue of antibiotics."

"That's right."

I then called West-One before leaving and left a message for Dr. Kravitz to get back to me.

The last time I had seen Dr. Melner, all I could do for forty minutes was sit across from him and sob. This time, I raged. I sat on the edge of the chair, tense and strained, and in a semicoherent manner described the mess we were in.

"They're all cowards. They know what they're doing is wrong. They know Andrea should be spared their interventions, that she is dying. They're afraid to let her go, to risk an investigation from God knows where. We're stuck, and I will either lose my mind or. . . . I think of suing the hospital, but where would that get us in a society of cowards, in a society that considers death the ultimate enemy?'' I railed at everyone at every level of opposition that I had thus far encountered, from Dr. Stein to judges on the Missouri Supreme Court.

"And I had this macabre exchange with Kathy about possible ways she might die, you know, how we can get around the feeding tube, which way would be quicker, pneumonia or I don't know what. . . . I think maybe I should find someone with the flu to go see her and cough all over her. . . . And her eyes are open: a nurse said her eyes have opened." I paused to stifle a wave of sadness. I didn't want to feel it. I preferred the anger. "And to top it off, every fucking week we get bills from doctors we've never heard of. I'll tell you, at this point I either throw them away or stuff them in some folder and forward it to the lawyer."

"Deborah," he interjected, "are you sleeping? Are you eating?"

"Not too well. I'm tense. I could use a tranquilizer," I admitted reluctantly.

"Have you ever used Valium?"

"Yeah. That might help." I felt ashamed to request medication to calm me down. I minimized the stress I was under, but weight loss, insomnia, and activated colitis belied my efforts to stay cool.

Right after the session Dr. Melner had me see his internist, whose office was in the neighborhood, to get a prescription. Following an overall physical exam, the doctor and I talked a bit. After hearing more about my predicament, he expressed dismay over the government's increasing interference in his profession. He couldn't even give me Valium, he said, without using a special form that went onto a data base in Albany. "My rights as a doctor, my job as a physician, are undermined by regulations," he complained. Then he added, "Sweden, I believe, has legalized euthanasia."

"How do we get Andrea there?" I asked.

Back at the apartment, there was a phone message from Kravitz. I called immediately and, amazingly enough, got him. He confirmed the nurse's report that Andrea's eyes were indeed open "and staring." This, he said, was not a good sign. From what I was beginning to understand, this meant that she was going from a comatose state (with eyes closed) to a persistent vegetative one that would last the duration of her life.

"Dr. Kravitz, if Andrea gets an infection, would antibiotics be administered?"

"Well, we have to wait until something happens, and I'd have to confer with my colleagues."

"What I'm asking is if Andrea develops an infection, could you *not* give her antibiotics? Is this possible?"

"Mrs. Alecson, we know how you feel about it, and we'll try to make it come out right."

"What does that mean?"

"We would not be as aggressive as with some other patients."

I couldn't get a straight answer. He said he had to do rounds before leaving for the day and that he'd be willing to discuss the matter further at another time.

My last call of the evening was to Dr. Minsky. Though loyal to the midwives and Dr. Kembel, having been the pediatrician for many of the babies they had brought into the world, he was also genuinely concerned for Andrea and for Lowell and me. Of Andrea's condition he said, "It's not a fatal illness, and it's not life." He appreciated our dilemma but did not know of any placements for her.

Then Kathy called to report that she had been unable to find a placement for Andrea. I had to give Lowell the phone because I started to cry and couldn't stop.

Lowell and I went to bed that night very aware that it had been six days since we had last seen Andrea. We had never actually planned to stop seeing her; we just took it day by day. As her fate, which certainly included treatment decisions and future long-term placements, became further out of our control, we followed our instincts, and these dictated that we maintain a distance. An intuitive self-preservation guided our actions. We knew that to cope, to carry on with our lives, to attempt to get what we wanted for her, we had to stay away from West-One. For me, I knew, to see her would plunge me into such despair that my impulse to save her from life, to kill her myself, would be rekindled. This impulse, this collision of maternal desires, would sooner destroy me than her.

Before falling asleep, we talked.

"Lowell, I have this belief that by not seeing Andrea, I will help her to die. It may just be magical thinking, but abandoned babies, babies who receive no physical contact, babies deprived of warmth, die. They die from lack of human warmth. Do you think this is bizarre?"

"No, I believe that's possible."

"Maybe I'm just rationalizing so that I won't feel guilty about not seeing her. But I don't think so. If we let her go, she'll let go."

"We can only hope."

I spent most of Wednesday reading *Playing God in the Nursery*. I learned that the original Baby Doe regulations were revised by Dr. C. Everett Koop because the American Academy of Pediatrics, the National Association of Children's Hospitals, and the Children's Hospital National Medical Center in Washington questioned their legality. On April

14, 1983, U.S. District Court Judge Gerhard Gesell deemed the regulations unacceptable as written.

Before the new regulations went into effect, a baby, later to be known as Baby Jane Doe, was born on October 11, 1983, with multiple birth defects on Long Island. Any one of the many physical and mental abnormalities she suffered should have been enough reason to withhold life support. After much consideration, the parents decided to forgo the corrective surgery that would have prolonged her life but would have offered minimal physical improvement. They requested that the baby be kept comfortable, fed, and treated with antibiotics if necessary (unlike the first Baby Doe).

The doctors concurred. However, one person (and that's all it takes) at the hospital disagreed and called an attorney representing the right-to-life movement in Vermont. This man, A. Lawrence Washburn, never saw Baby Jane Doe, never spoke to the parents or to the doctors, yet he took it upon himself to defend the rights of the "handicapped" child (as he had done many times before). He filed in New York for a court order to have the surgery done. A court hearing followed, with testimony from medical specialists, pleas from right-to-life advocates—and further misery for the parents.

Justice Melvyn Tanenbaum ruled that the surgery must be performed to ensure the infant's survival. The lawyer for the parents appealed, whereupon Justice Lawrence Bracken of the Appellate Division reversed Tanenbaum's decision.

A. Lawrence Washburn appealed to New York's highest court, the Court of Appeals, which upheld the appellate court's decision. Responding to complaints from the American Life Lobby, a right-to-life organization, the Reagan administration ultimately stepped in. The Department of

Health and Human Services demanded the baby's records in order to determine whether the hospital was in violation of federal regulations—specifically, section 504 of the Rehabilitation Act of 1973.

The Rehabilitation Act of 1973 insures civil rights to the handicapped in employment and housing. Section 504 forbids discrimination based on disability by those institutions receiving federal funds. The Reagan administration thus hoped to apply this act to the withholding of medical treatment for imperiled newborns in hospitals receiving federal monies.

While reading Jeff Lyon's account I was struck by this line, and marked it in my book: "The immense power of the federal government was being used to bully one lonely couple, already engulfed in personal sorrow" (p. 51).

I had to absorb all this information in small doses. The involvement of so many people completely outside the intimate struggle of this family to accept their child's devastation and to stand by their decision regarding her treatment infuriated me. It was beyond my understanding how some guy in Vermont could go out of his way to push for an ideology of what was right and what was wrong in his own mind, at the expense of humane consideration for this severely deformed infant and her family. This man was not responsible for the conception of this child. This man did not carry this child for nine months. And this man would not witness, day in and day out, the impoverishment of this child's existence. He wouldn't deal with her pain and suffering. He wouldn't deal with the medical bills. He wouldn't bury her after her tortured life on earth was over.

On Thursday, June 29, I turned thirty-five. That morning, I hadn't the wherewithal to celebrate, but the evening before, in a moment of normal sentiments, I had yielded to Lowell's enthusiasm to do something special and we made a reservation for dinner aboard a yacht. My last two birth-days had been celebrated in this way, though at thirty-four I was recuperating from the miscarriage and feeling empty and sad. Little did I know then that that blighted hope would seem like small potatoes compared to what I'd be experiencing on the next anniversary of my birth. While pregnant with Andrea I had expected to have the greatest of all birthday presents: my own baby girl, nursing in my arms. The pang of that shattered vision was all I could feel as I faced the day.

Fortunately, I had scheduled an afternoon therapy ses-sion. I walked into Dr. Melner's office and announced, "I feel more depressed, if that's possible, than the last time I saw you." We decided that the Valium might be partly to blame, so Dr. Melner suggested I try the antidepressant Prozac.

This time I did not carry on about spineless doctors, or rant and rave about right-to-life advocates. This time I cried. I felt utterly hopeless and defeated.

"Last night I talked to Kathy, the doctor from the Has-tings Center, about placements, and she said she'd had no luck finding one. She also suggested that we ask the ethics committee to discuss antibiotics, to get the hospital not to give Andrea any if she should develop an infection. I started sobbing on the phone and had to put Lowell on."

Dr. Melner, who had always known just what to say during all those past therapy sessions, before Andrea, in which I exposed my familial pain and pieced together one broken connection after another, was uncustomarily silent. What could he say? God Himself would not know what to say.

I didn't need to hear him talk anyway. I just needed to feel. Dr. Melner provided me with a safe place in which to purge myself. I had done so little crying that week that my sorrow poured out, and every so often I would find the right words. "I was tortured last night by my urge to see her," I admitted, as if it was a debased desire.

Yes, that was what was at the core.

As I left Dr. Melner's office he gave me a hug and said, "Happy Birthday."

Dressed for once in something other than my brown dress—a sky blue sleeveless and cleavage-revealing summer knit—we made our way to the Hudson River dock at Twenty-third Street to board the ship. It was a sparkling clear evening of warm breezes, with a fiery sun setting in the west. My emotions changed swiftly like a sky that suddenly darkens then brightens as clouds sweep across the sun; one minute I felt the airy excitement of the occasion, and the next, the crushing weight of despair.

We got ourselves settled at our table by the piano, where a woman sang and accompanied herself. Lowell had performed in this manner at parties and special events, and we both listened and commented on her performance. Before sailing, a waiter approached to ask if we wanted cocktails; after some deliberation, we went ahead and ordered champagne. To make even that gesture toward honoring myself, though, was a heavyhearted concession.

With our champagne before us and a toast to be made, we slowly left Manhattan behind. Surrounding us were gay and satisfied diners treating themselves to an exceptional evening of eating and drinking, dancing, and the enthralling sight of a diminishing and luminous New York City. Lowell and I clinked glasses. "Here's to my Baby Face on her birthday," he said. I started to cry.

"I'm sorry. This was a mistake," I said, muffling my sobs so as not to call attention to myself. I got up and went to the bathroom, where I stood before a mirror and looked directly into my face for several minutes. "Deborah," I scolded myself, "Lowell is trying very hard to bring us above our unhappiness and to have us enjoy one night out. Pull yourself together, if not for your sake, then for his." After this speech to my reflection, I returned to our table, where the hors d'oeuvre was waiting.

Lowell presented me with earrings. They were as beautiful as they were extravagant, but after trying them on I decided that I'd prefer a more modest and casual pair that I could wear on a regular basis. Lowell accepted this graciously; we had always been able to negotiate the gifts we bought each other and concede to differing tastes.

Lowell, valiant and loving throughout the night, kept me as buoyant as was humanly possible. We even danced a few slow numbers, an extended embrace as we glided across the floor. Standing out on the deck, watching the bejeweled city continually transform as we navigated the river, I felt the world expand beyond my personal sorrow. It was a welcome perspective.

The next day, after exchanging the earrings and getting my wedding rings polished in Chinatown's diamond district, I wrote in my journal:

> While in the jewelry shop I found myself unable to make
> an aesthetic judgment. I couldn't tell what looked nice
> or what looked good on me. It is a problem I have with
> clothing as well, and the situation seems to be getting
> worse. I also picked up a new bathing suit to replace the
> rag I've been wearing, only to find that I need a size
> smaller. But I couldn't tell if it really fit, and I needed the
> feedback of the old shlub who works there. This all must
> be a part of my depression. I can't really tell if food tastes
> good or what to choose to eat, so I eat the same things,
> or not at all.
>
> Choice itself is difficult to deal with.

Dr. Melner had said that it takes a few weeks before Prozac kicks in. But I was beginning to conclude that my depression was normal and should not be inhibited, unless I became totally nonfunctional; so I stopped taking the drug. Not knowing how to attire myself to my best advantage was a far cry from not being able to get dressed at all. True, I had tried and retried the exact same bathing suit in three different sizes for an inordinate length of time before trusting myself to buy one. Yet at least I was capable of recognizing that the bathing suit I had been wearing was in tatters, and I did have enough self-esteem to want to look presentable at the pool. I wasn't that far gone.

Soon Independence Day weekend was upon us, and Lowell and I passed it by visiting different members of my family. On Saturday we went to The Farm, where we saw not only my parents, but also my sister, her husband, and their two children. My reaction to seeing my niece took me by surprise: I hadn't anticipated such sadness and envy.

We spent Sunday with my mother at Brighton Beach in Brooklyn, where we swam in the ocean, lay on the sand, and looked longingly at children with pails and shovels at play by the shore. It was becoming apparent that seeing children, even our own relatives, made us ache; and we noticed children, wherever we went, more than ever.

On our way back to Manhattan we paid a spontaneous visit to my grandparents, who were still recuperating from the bus accident. My grandmother was ensconced in a living-room chair with her legs up. We talked while I rubbed her feet with Mineral Ice.

"All I want is to be able to walk," she said.

"Grandma, you just had an operation for a broken hip. You'll walk. It takes time to heal."

She had had eighty-five robust years, and the few times

she did have minor ailments she would see her son, my
uncle the chiropractor, who would give her an adjustment
and send her home. I noticed how attentive my grandparents were to each other, more demonstrative than I had
ever seen. They no longer seemed to take each other for
granted; a mutual appreciation had been renewed.

"It's wonderful what trauma can do for a marriage," I
commented to Lowell on the subway as we returned to
Manhattan.

That evening we called West-One before dinner. We were
told that Andrea was in a crib and that she had had a fever
all weekend. The nurse was unable to tell us the cause. My
resolve not to see her collapsed.

"Lowell," I pleaded, "I've got to see her. I can't stay
away any longer. The need to see her is overwhelming me.
Will you come with me after dinner?"

"Are you sure, Deborah?"

"Yes, it's making me crazy."

"Okay. We'll see her after we eat."

As we were about to head out the door we stopped in the
kitchen to embrace, then kiss.

We never made it to the hospital. I lay in bed after our
lovemaking and wept as Lowell held me.

In the morning, Andrea still had a fever and needed a lot
of suctioning. The nurse said she was "quieter," whatever
that meant, and that her eyes were open but not focused.

I called Kathy and asked if she would speak with Dr.
Kravitz to find out how they planned to treat the fever.

Another medical probability was now weighing on our
minds. Way back when, a few days after the meeting with
Dr. Maslin and the others regarding the results of the neurological exams, Dr. Hines had asked me if we would consent
to a gastrostomy. He had asked me this in the hallway of the
NICU when I was there visiting Andrea, and all I could do

in response was inspect his face for irony. I thought, "I can't believe that this man is asking me for permission to insert a feeding tube directly into Andrea's stomach after my incessant pleas to have all the feedings stopped, nasogastric and IV. Have we been talking the same language? Has he not understood a single thing I've said in all this time?" After I regained my senses I said slowly, "We would never consent to a gastrostomy. Never."

He replied, "I thought that's how you felt."

The idea of a gastrostomy was being raised again because Andrea couldn't tolerate feedings through the nose and she often had to be suctioned. I imagined that it would make life easier for the NICU staff to have a tube through which liquid nutrition could be poured into her stomach directly, bypassing the respiratory tract. A gastrostomy would also reduce the possibility of infection. So far, we had been able to oppose it, but it was conceivable that the hospital would try to get a court order to have it done.

The prospect of a gastrostomy drove us to call Lowell's mother's cousin Erik, in Denmark. We asked Erik if he would find out about the laws in Denmark, Sweden, Norway, and the Netherlands regarding euthanasia and hospice care for impaired newborns. It was an outrageous path to take, but we felt desperate. We followed up our call with a letter that described the circumstances of Andrea's birth and her current medical status.

It was only later in the day, when I spoke with Ricky, that I realized the near impossibility of bringing this alternative to actualization. As Ricky pointed out, "You'd need a court order to transfer her to another country." Kathy, to whom I also presented the scheme, explained that the adverse effects of transporting her would necessitate more medical intervention. That was something we did not want.

We were back to plan A: getting the doctors not to give

Andrea antibiotics. Kathy suggested that we might need to make a tradeoff: consenting to the gastrostomy if they promised not to treat her should an infection develop.

Notwithstanding what Dr. Cassell believed, we felt as if Andrea was being held hostage and we had to bargain for her release.

8

Acceptance

Playing God in the Nursery continued to give me a context for understanding Andrea's place both in the NICU and in the national conscience. She was caught in a web of political policies that immobilized everyone concerned. What I read made me angry, but it also helped me to see our personal sorrow as something that went beyond Dr. Stein, Dr. Hines, and even the dreaded hospital lawyers. At the same time, I came to realize that we were all in this mess together.

According to Jeff Lyon's account, one of the judges on the New York Court of Appeals shared my outrage at A. Lawrence Washburn's meddling, stating: "How come a perfect stranger can interfere in the family decisions in a tragic situation such as this?" (p. 50).

The government's lawsuit against the hospital, which claimed the right to examine Baby Jane Doe's medical records, was ruled on by U.S. District Court Judge Leonard D. Wexler on Long Island on November 17, 1983. He pronounced that section 504 of the 1973 Rehabilitation Act was not violated in this case because the hospital had been willing to perform the surgery if the parents had requested it. Furthermore, the parents' decision not to make such a request was found to be reasonable given the condition of their baby and the prognosis.

The government appealed, only to be cut down again on February 23, 1984, when the U.S. Court of Appeals affirmed Judge Wexler's ruling. Moreover, it ruled that the intent of section 504 was to insure equality in housing and employment, not to make hospitals employ heroic measures for every damaged baby born within their walls. The revised Baby Doe regulations were therefore held to be invalid. As a result of this ruling, the Department of Health and Human Services no longer had the authority to investigate hospitals.

This wasn't the end of the story, though. Congress passed the 1984 Child Abuse Amendments to the Child Abuse and Treatment and Adoption Reform Act of 1974. The amendments, signed into law by Ronald Reagan on October 9, 1984, assured the medical treatment of handicapped children. Child abuse was redefined to include the withholding of medical treatment from children whose lives were threatened by their physical condition. Exceptions were allowed, however, including the nontreatment of an infant deemed to be comatose. But this nontreatment did not encompass the withholding of nutrition and hydration.

What I found so insensible about this legislation was that it disregarded the quality of life a severely damaged infant might be expected to have. Moreover, doctors and hospitals, faced with the task of interpreting the laws and their application to the newborns in their care, never knew for certain whether or not they were in compliance. Consequently, the safest course of action was always to treat every impaired newborn to the utmost.

"How does this affect *us?*" I wondered after a morning of reading.

Andrea fit the exceptions to the rule: she was comatose, she was dying, her damage was irreversible, and there was no treatment that could correct her condition. However, we weren't fighting the hospital on whether or not to perform a surgical procedure or to take her off a respirator. We were requesting that she not be fed, which goes straight to the heart of what it is to act humanely toward others in their living and in their dying. We were trespassing in the realm of religious beliefs, taboos, and gut reactions. Furthermore, starving a baby to death was infanticide.

I concluded that when Drs. Cassell, Nolan, and Stein mentioned the Baby Doe regs, they were really referring to a political attitude of medical conservatism in the country. The original regulations and the revised version no longer existed, but the laws passed by Congress that broadened the definition of child abuse, and the aftereffects of the Baby Doe regulations, had created an atmosphere of excessive caution. Doctors now strove always to save and prolong life rather than allow the natural dying process to prevail in some cases.

As I was preparing to go for a swim, Kathy called. "I had a very good talk with Dr. Kravitz," she said. "I feel he is on your side."

"Which means?"

"I believe he recognizes that what you and Lowell want for Andrea is right."

I had already sensed this, but it didn't seem to make any difference when it came to his actions.

"Did you ask him about her fever and antibiotics?"

"Yes. Her fever is either due to an infection or due to a neurological impairment that makes her body incapable of maintaining a normal temperature. Dr. Kravitz is treating the fever as a symptom of her neurological damage, for which there is no cure.''

''I don't understand. How does this relate to whether or not she'll be getting antibiotics?''

''If it's assumed that she doesn't have an infection, she won't be given antibiotics.''

''What do you think will happen?''

''I think Dr. Kravitz will let nature take its course without intervening.''

''Thank you so much for talking to him and for sharing this with me.''

After a pause she said, ''Deborah, I really think you and Lowell will get what you want for Andrea, but it may not be in the way you want, in the time you want. This is very delicate, and there are many considerations besides your urgent need to have your daughter spared.''

Before we hung up, I asked her if she was a Buddhist. She sounded pleased that I was able to determine what her religion was. I figured it out based on my understanding of Buddhist doctrine and on things she had said that gave me the impression that she viewed death as another stage of life, and life as a state of impermanence.

My driving desire had been to set Andrea free, and I had believed that her freedom was to be found in her death. Now, for the first time since her birth, I realized that she didn't have to die to be free. She already was free. Who Andrea was, her essence, was not to be found in her body. Instead, it was I who was not free. I had been struggling with my attachment to the child she should have been and to my overpowering longing to be her mother, to fulfill that destiny.

My revelation was interrupted by the phone. It was a woman from the Hemlock Society in Los Angeles. I gave her a synopsis of our situation but she told me that her organization did not deal with babies. I was disappointed that Derek Humphry himself had not returned my call.

At the club, I ran into Serena, a woman I had become friendly with when I was in my first trimester with Andrea. She knew what had happened, and we had spoken by phone occasionally since the birth. At some point during our poolside conversation she asked, ''What's the matter? You seem upset.'' Her question was so disconcerting that I concluded she must have had led a life free from catastrophe; either that, or she was really obtuse. Whichever it was, I felt there was a limit to what I could share with her and expect her to grasp. Then she told me about a woman she knew named Jeanie who, with her four-month-old daughter, Kelly, was in a situation similar to mine. I asked Serena for her phone number.

When I got back to my apartment, I sat before the phone for several minutes before calling Jeanie. What should I say? Where to begin? How do you talk about such things? What if she *doesn't* talk about it, and my call only upset her?

Jeanie answered the phone; the first thing I heard was a weariness in her voice. But she was more than willing to talk, relieved to have found someone who was going through the same thing.

Kelly had been born brain damaged, without a corpus callosum and brain tissue was missing in both her hemispheres. Jeanie had gone into premature labor, and after weeks of taking a drug to control her contractions, the baby was born three weeks early. This wasn't the cause of the brain damage; it was the result of it. Like many fetuses that are malformed, it had been trying to abort itself. In the not too distant past, the baby either would have been stillborn or would have died soon after birth. But Jeanie was in a hospital, and modern medicine intervened.

"It wasn't until I brought her to a hospital in Boston to be checked out when she was a month old that I found out she was brain damaged."

"What do you mean?"

"The doctors in the intensive care unit at the hospital where she was born didn't tell us anything. I thought she was sick and would get better. The first time I heard the words 'brain damage' was in Boston."

"Didn't they do tests?"

"Yes, and they must not have found anything. The CAT scan they did just didn't pick it up."

I told her about our suspicions from day one that Andrea had sustained brain damage because of asphyxiation. "For us, it was a question of how much."

During that first month, she and her husband had consented to a gastrostomy because Kelly's esophagus was damaged and she was vomiting and choking all the time when she was fed. This surgery saved her life. After they had learned of the extent of her brain damage, they asked that the G-tube be removed. The hospital refused. Even with the G-tube, Jeanie didn't expect Kelly to live long.

"We found a placement for her in the city, and she'll be transferred this month," she said.

She told me that she visits Kelly for two hours every single day after work, and all day Saturday and Sunday.

"Your husband too?"

"No. He's dealing with this differently. He will have nothing to do with Kelly." Her tone of voice revealed the strain her marriage was under.

I felt overwhelming compassion for her.

"Have you ever considered not seeing her?" I asked.

"Absolutely not."

"Why?"

"Because I have to," she answered.

I wanted to tell her, "Let go—give her up, get on with your life."

"Six weeks after Kelly's birth I was a basket case, unable to talk to anyone about what was going on. I'm amazed that you can, that you seem so stable."

"Believe me, I have periods when I'm devastated. I'm hoping that if I stay away from Andrea, she will die. That may sound strange, but it's how I feel."

We talked a little more. I suspected that she felt I was abandoning my daughter; and I thought she was sacrificing her life, and perhaps her marriage, for hers. After we hung up, I felt grateful to have created more distance within a month and a half than she had in four. Jeanie had thought Kelly would recover; for that reason, the claims on her life were stronger. I'd had to come to terms with Andrea's condition immediately; my bonding with her had always been tenuous.

I reflected on our conversation for quite some time. My sympathy was more for Jeanie than for Kelly. It was the same pity I had felt for myself, the self I had been when I, too, felt compelled to see my baby. I believed that Jeanie's sympathy, however, was for Andrea, not for me, and for all the babies she saw neglected at the hospital where Kelly was kept.

Our talk stirred up a lot. I could now understand how others must have felt listening to me during those early days when I was engulfed. I so wanted Jeanie to let go, just as others had wanted me to let go. But at that time, my life was secondary to Andrea's. It was Andrea's pain that mattered. It was Andrea's existence that had to be considered, not mine, not Lowell's. Jeanie (like me, during those fragile first weeks) had no choice but to put her unresponsive, unknowing, unaware baby at the very center of her life.

For the rest of the afternoon and into the night, I questioned the meaning of devotion. Jeanie and I were clearly handling things differently. I was not visiting Andrea, whereas she was seeing Kelly whenever she could. At one time I would have said that she was a better mother than I, that she was more devoted. Now I wondered, "To whom is she devoted?"

On Saturday morning, Lowell and I packed for a two-week stay at The Farm. My father and stepmother were taking a vacation and had invited us to house-sit, to take advantage of their spacious home and be miles away from the city and from the hospital. Since I had doctor appointments on Monday and Lowell had voice lessons scheduled all week, we planned to go up for the weekend, return Sunday evening, then I'd go back upstate for the rest of the time my parents would be gone. Lowell would either commute back and forth or stay in the city, depending on his schedule.

Kitty and I had spoken on the telephone Friday morning before they were to leave. She told me where to find various booklets about the appliances in the house, she described how the fuse box worked, she gave me the names and phone numbers of their plumber, electrician, etcetera—and she had me take down the name of an undertaker we could call if Andrea should die while they were away.

"All you'll have to do is make one phone call, and everything will be taken care of," she said.

Up until that moment, I hadn't considered what we would do when Andrea died. Lowell and I had never discussed it. We'd certainly talked enough about allowing her to die, but we never actually talked about what we would do with her corpse, or whether we'd have a funeral. Kitty's investigation into morticians seemed premature to me; even during my most despairing moments, I'd had it fixed in my mind that Andrea would go on forever and ever. The possibility that she might die in the next few weeks was unimaginable.

My parents, however—thorough, organized, always prepared—had made arrangements because they felt Lowell and I would appreciate not having to do so when the time came. I did not believe that the time would ever come, that the doctors would have the courage to let Andrea slip away—despite Kathy's view of Dr. Kravitz's position.

Along with two weeks' worth of clothes and paraphernalia, we packed Andrea's things. We would store the contents of the nursery as well as my pregnancy clothes at The Farm. Rattles, teething rings, plastic balls, and stuffed animals went into one bag. Nursing supplies—pads, the plastic pump, funnels, bottles, nipples—went into another. Then I stuffed the bags into separate compartments of the changing table. Lowell dismantled the cradle and carried the parts downstairs to my parents' van (on loan), which was parked in front of our building.

We didn't linger over the items, not even the special gifts we had received for Andrea at the shower. We left her baby clothes in the drawers of the dresser we had painted especially for her pleasure, and hauled each drawer separately, that Ivory Snow baby smell still strongly scenting the air. It was with a dislocated faith that I folded my maternity dresses, jumpers, and stretch pants. I couldn't begin to imagine being pregnant again, wearing those same clothes, outfitted for a wholly new life inside.

It was the square flowered box of tissues that did me in. It was open, one pink tissue beckoning to be plucked. I didn't know whether or not to save it, that box of broken dreams. I began to sob. Then I used the tissue to wipe my eyes and packed the box inside the changing table.

With great optimism, we also transported Lowell's electric piano, trusting that he would have the spirit to play and sing, to give voice to all that he had been keeping restrained. Lowell lugged the computer and printer he had borrowed from the high school for the summer. Maybe I'd be moved to compose a poem, to find the language that could begin to express all that I felt.

Before walking out the door, I called the NICU to leave our phone number upstate. I spoke with a nurse named Elizabeth, who reported, "Andrea can't control her own temperature, so we've put on additional clothing to keep her warm, and blankets."

"Where is she?"

"In a crib."

"Are her eyes open?" It was a question I asked, though it tortured me to do so.

"They're open halfway. We've been putting drops in her eyes every six hours."

"Okay, thank you. I just wanted you all to know where we can be reached."

As I put down the receiver, I visualized her sweet little face, the hazel irises of her eyes peeking through lowered lids like two flags at half-mast.

During the ride upstate, I told Lowell about my phone conversation with Kitty and her arrangements with an undertaker. "She said all we'd have to do is make one phone call. You know, you and I never talked about any of that. First of all, I can't even imagine Andrea being dead. What do you think?"

"About her being dead, or about the undertaker?"

"About how we'd handle it. What you would want. You know—a funeral."

"I don't know. I'd have to think about it. I would want her cremated. I would want myself cremated, so I certainly would want her cremated. Do you agree?"

"Yes. And I'm pretty sure that I wouldn't want a funeral."

We both fell silent. Looking out the window of the van I added, "I don't know, maybe I'll feel different when the time comes."

And we said no more about it.

After a weekend of settling in at The Farm, I passed a busy Monday of doctor appointments in the city. My periodontist found my gums to be in excellent shape. He expressed his sorrow at what we were going through and, shaking his head, remarked, "I've told people I know about what happened to you, mostly other doctors, and they all agreed that it is practically unheard of that a baby should be born in your daughter's condition. It is a terrible, terrible thing."

From his office I went to Dr. Gilmer for a gynecological exam. The last time I had seen her was when I responded to her question, "How can I help you?" by unleashing a torrent of tears. She now determined that my uterus had shrunk as it should have, and she suggested that I forgo birth control in mid-August if I wanted to get pregnant. I told her that we were engaged in a malpractice lawsuit, to which she replied, "I'm not one to encourage malpractice lawsuits, but in your case I believe there has been liability." She went on to say, "Anyone can deliver a baby. Taxi drivers deliver babies. It is the ten percent of complicated labors that need the expertise of a doctor."

"Do you think if I should get pregnant again, I could try for a vaginal birth?" The thought of going through another Caesarean section was more than I could bear.

"I don't see why not."

"Why, then, was I laboring for all those hours, with fierce contractions, and the baby wouldn't descend?"

"It could very well have been because of her position," she said. "I recently delivered a baby vaginally for a woman who had to have Caesarean sections for both her other children. It's a matter of position."

I walked out of her office feeling consumed with remorse that I hadn't listened to Rhonda and used Dr. Gilmer to deliver Andrea. If only, if only, if only . . .

Lowell was to remain in the city until Thursday, when I'd come in to meet him for a joint therapy session and we'd return upstate together. Monday evening, alone on the train to Brewster, I wondered about the upcoming days when I'd be isolated in the country with plenty of time and few distractions. I felt anxious about how I'd handle the emotions that would surely surface while I was by myself. But I also knew that I needed solitude in order to make sense of my feelings about Andrea: her reality versus my idea of who she was and who she could have become. I wanted to call on nature to give me the kind of perspective that I could not get in the city. I needed to know that I had the inner resources to achieve a sense of well-being, a sense of hope for my future life. But first I had to get in touch with my deepest regrets and my most profound fears if Andrea should live. I had to feel my sorrow unrestrained and then return to myself.

After a dinner of cold cooked chicken and wilted salad that I found in the refrigerator, I walked around the grounds of my parent's property as evening descended. Gradually, one by one, stars emerged from the darkening sky, until a blanket of them glistened above. I stretched out on my back on the slanting lawn and stared into the night. I listened to the chirping of crickets and the rhythmic droning of cicadas. And I waited. I waited for an insight into the disaster of Andrea.

I watched fireflies flickering on and off and the headlights and taillights of cars disappearing down roads in the distance. It wasn't long before I attracted a cluster of mosquitoes, which savagely attacked my exposed flesh. Insight did not come before I sought shelter indoors from those bloodthirsty insects; but tears did, and I sat cross-legged, grabbing the earth in my fists, and cried.

Before going to bed, I called Lowell to say goodnight.

"I miss you," I said.

"I miss you too," he replied.

"Sleep well. I love you."

"I love you too."

For the next few days I got into a routine of an early-morning walk along dirt roads and an afternoon workout in an outdoor pool belonging to a friend of my parents', who also was away. Putting *Playing God in the Nursery* aside, I started to read *The Road Less Traveled* by M. Scott Peck because of its first line: "Life is difficult." With that beginning I counted on a book that would tell me something I didn't already know, or remind me of what I always knew but had forgotten.

At six A.M., the coolest part of the day, I would put on my running shoes and cross the dew-covered lawn until I reached the gravel driveway that led to an unpaved road. While I walked, I thought about Andrea. At three in the afternoon, after the hottest hours had peaked, I swam laps in the neighbor's pool, and thought about Andrea. I was beginning to accept that I had done everything I could for her. Throughout it all, I still believed in the universal justice of nature. I also maintained a faith that, if nothing else, lack of human contact and maternal nurturing would hasten her death.

I still had moments, agonizing moments, when I wanted to see her. I realized that it was a masochistic impulse, a need to punish myself for what had happened, and that seeing her would not make her better; it would only annihilate me. Furthermore, what there was in the NICU lying under those blankets was not Andrea, but her shell. She was more present to me in my thoughts, as I walked the country roads and gazed at the stars, than she could ever be as a vacant doll, immobile in a crib before me.

One afternoon, with great trepidation, I sat at a typewriter and wrote a poem to Lowell. The first stanza came to me at once:

> Our love fused in my womb grew
> as microscopic matter and
> the imaginings of our minds.

By the time I finished the poem, I was sobbing. I had said all that I had to say at that moment; with the words found and the poem complete, I felt my sorrow lighten.

On Wednesday afternoon, Lowell called to say that he was catching the 7:08 to Brewster North and we could drive into the city together the next morning for our session. I was delighted.

Reunited, we dined outside on the deck and drank the bottle of champagne we had bought to celebrate Andrea's birth. Lowell, though practically a teetotaler, suggested that another bottle was in order and drove off to town to pick one up while I cleared the table of dishes.

Next to the deck was a small oval pool, so well secluded from nearby houses that skinny-dipping could be privately enjoyed, even in broad daylight. After we'd polished off the second bottle, Lowell suddenly undressed and plunged into the water; I quickly followed. It was precisely this kind of organic spontaneity that I needed, something we could never have had in Manhattan. We splashed and frolicked as the sun set, finally falling into each other's arms, exhilarated and exhausted.

Thursday afternoon, Lowell and I found ourselves seated side by side on a couch, holding hands, facing Susan Atkins, a therapist we had seen once the previous week. Before us was a large round glass table displaying amethyst formations and assorted geological gems. The last time, among other feelings, we had discussed my ambivalence about not seeing Andrea.

"How are you both doing?" she asked.

Lowell and I looked at each other, then I answered, "Well, we haven't been seeing Andrea."

"And how has that been?"

"For me," I said, "every day it gets a little easier to stay away, though I do have spells when I feel a desperate urge to see her. Instead, I call West-One, and the report is always that her temperature can't be regulated and that she needs a lot of suctioning. I think the doctor now in charge wants her to be allowed to die and is looking for a way to let it happen without getting into trouble."

"It sounds like you're preparing yourselves for that, for her death. How do you do that? How do you say goodbye?"

Again, Lowell and I looked at each other. He started to cry, and I put my arms around him. He embraced me, and we stayed that way, intertwined, until he gained composure.

"It's still so hard to believe that this is all happening," he said, reaching for my hand, "but I think we have to let go of her."

After a silence, Susan asked, "Have you always adored each other, or has this tragedy brought it out?"

"We've been pretty lucky with each other," Lowell answered.

As we left her office questions remained: How do we say goodbye? What ritual must we create?

At The Farm, we prepared for a five-day visit from our friends Arthur and Lyla, whose wedding we had attended when I was in my first trimester with Andrea. Regardless of the emotional ups and downs Lowell and I were experiencing, we believed that it was possible for us all to find pleasure in one another's company.

I was in my bathing suit sitting on a chaise longue by the

side of the pool when Lyla and Arthur's car pulled up the driveway. It was a hot, sunny Saturday afternoon; waving in greeting, I yelled, "Get your bathing suits on." As they approached, I felt momentarily self-conscious of my post-pregnant figure. Lyla was eight years my junior and voluptuous, svelte though generously endowed, with thick dark hair that fell in waves around her lovely face and shoulders. While I had never possessed a flat stomach, I now had one that folded vertically in the middle; I was sure the whole world could see that mammoth incision right through my clothes. The first words out of Arthur's mouth were, "You look great." I replied, "Thank you. I guess I'm looking all right for an old gal who just had a baby."

Unfortunately, the sun went into hiding for the remainder of their stay, so instead of relaxing by the pool, we went for car rides in search of historical sites and bookstores, took walks when the weather permitted, and stayed inside discussing art, politics, marriage, and, of course, Andrea. They knew bits and pieces about the circumstances of her birth and all that followed, but one rainy afternoon we presented the whole story. Lyla listened intently to everything we said, asking questions and encouraging us to talk about our feelings.

"You guys have been through so much, and you're both so strong. I don't know how I would handle it," she said.

For Arthur, it was more difficult to just listen. He needed to talk about himself and his struggle as an aspiring writer; it wasn't easy for him to be receptive to our situation, which was so different from his own. As a consequence, Lowell and I grew closer to Lyla, eventually learning of her unhappiness with Arthur.

One early evening as Lyla cooked dinner for us all (we were taking turns putting meals together), I was moved to write a poem to Andrea. I excused myself and retreated to the study, leaving Arthur to his reading and Lowell to the piano.

Seated before the typewriter, I realized that *this* was my way of saying goodbye, *this* was my ritual. Halfway through the poem I wrote:

> My darling little girl,
> I am dumb to explain your fate,
> powerless to stop what you've become:
> gone from your body
> that breathes to feign life.
>
> You are an innocent
> with a soul like a halo
> that encircles and waits
> to merge with your body.

The tears came, and, pressing on to completion, I had what I could only describe as a catharsis.

The morning of the day Lyla and Arthur were to leave, we all went for a long walk. The nature of their marital difficulties was further revealed. A central problem, it turned out, was money. They didn't have much of their own, and Arthur, who spent frivolously, asked for and accepted large sums from his father. Arthur's financial dependence upset Lyla, who believed it kept him a child. Now, after nearly a year of marriage, they maintained separate bank accounts. "I think this whole money thing is a symptom of something deeper, namely, a lack of trust in each other," I said, never being one to beat around the bush. I encouraged them to consider, as a first step, opening a joint account, though I had my reservations. I was worried for Lyla; from all that I had heard and witnessed during their stay, I wondered if Arthur had the discipline and maturity to save and to plan for their future together.

I listened to them talk about their creative endeavors as

artists (Lyla was an actress) and the support they needed from each other as they traveled their individual roads to acclaim. If Lyla got a role in a show that took her to Europe, she said, she would go. If Arthur's work took him to a writer's colony far away, he would go.

"You guys have to make your marriage the priority now, and not your artistic aspirations, otherwise there will always be conflict," I warned.

My advice to Lyla and Arthur made it seem as if Lowell and I had uncovered the secret of marital bliss after fifty years together. The fact was, we were practically newly-weds ourselves. Coping with Andrea and the immeasurable grief her limbo caused us had solidified the love and confidence we already had in each other. Besides, we simply did not have the emotional reserve to argue and disagree.

Before Lyla and Arthur left, I wanted to tell them that it wasn't career success or artistic glory that made life worth living or saw one through tough times. I wanted to tell them to invest in each other, to grow as lovers and friends, to make that their goal rather than social recognition of their talents. Instead, I bought them a copy of *The Road Less Traveled* and told them to read the section entitled "Love."

As Lowell and I stood watching Lyla and Arthur's car round the driveway and turn onto the road I said, "I don't think they're going to make it."

"Maybe, if they get some counseling," Lowell replied.

"I feel bad. I love them both, but I think that when they got married, Lyla made a commitment, while Arthur just went through the motions."

I could have continued talking about them, analyzing their relationship, but Lowell wasn't inclined to delve into other people's lives the way I was. He accepted people for what they were, while I scratched at surfaces expecting something truer to be exposed.

That evening, Lowell caught a late train into the city. He planned to take a yoga class at our health club first thing in the morning, and he had voice lessons to teach throughout the day. I was alone at The Farm once again. I needed the time, though, for we were expecting Lowell's parents, Tom and Edna, who were driving from Minnesota and planned to stay with us for at least a week. They were coming to see their new granddaughter.

The next morning I awoke to an inevitable yet unexpected surprise: my period had returned. I then figured out that if my cycle was as it had been before I was pregnant, I would probably be ovulating in August when we'd be at Kripalu, the yoga retreat where Andrea had been conceived a year ago. I didn't know if we'd be ready to try at that time, and I wondered about using that opportunity to do so. I had to be sure that my intention was not to replace Andrea or to recreate her. If I was to have another child, he or she would have to be born purely for his or her own sake. So much depended on what would happen in the next few months— whether Andrea would live, and whether a placement could be found for her.

Before setting out on a hike I called Dr. Kravitz, who reported, "Andrea remains the same." Then I spoke with Ricky about our case, and he said, "Further progress awaits evaluations from our medical experts." I checked in on my mother, who, on summer vacation from work, was spending her time on the beach near her apartment. We'd had frequent phone conversations over the weeks but hadn't seen much of each other. She had stopped visiting Andrea and was grieving.

As always since the day I was born, I had to make an effort to keep both my parents in my life. Resentments between them continued to thrive, and even Andrea, a shared heartbreak, could not abolish those old animosities. For my mother, my retreat to The Farm—my father's turf—created more than a physical distance between us.

"Mom, you're all right?" I asked before we hung up.

"I have good days and bad days. It's a process, letting go. I think about her a lot. Are you all right?"

"It's the same for me. I love you."

"I love you too, sweetheart."

"I'll call you when Lowell's parents arrive. Maybe we can all get together."

As I prepared for my walk I thought about the time I had called my mother, sobbing uncontrollably, and asked, "Will I ever experience joy again?" It was right after the ethics committee had changed its mind, and I felt tortured every minute of every hour by the image of Andrea being kept alive, tethered to a feeding machine in that unresponsive state, forever and ever. My mother had reassured me, "Yes, yes, you will have joy, in time." I didn't believe her. Now, tying the shoelaces of my sneakers, I acknowledged that a fragile ability to feel pleasure had returned. "I was so convinced, and not that long ago, that the ache would never go away, not even for an instant," I thought. Sunlight filtering through the leaves made patterns that danced along the dirt road as I made my way uphill. My tan cotton shorts and Lowell's white T-shirt became increasingly damp with perspiration as I climbed, anchoring a stick into the ground before each step. Every so often I would stop and listen to the trill of a breeze through the trees. For the first time since Andrea's birth, I felt a peace that could only have come from surrender.

Tom and Edna arrived Friday evening in time for a dinner of pizza and salad. They had never been to The Farm before, and as they approached the house, they exclaimed about the wonderful job my parents had done transforming an old barn and nine acres of property into an estate. While I organized our take-out dinner on the patio facing the pool, Lowell gave them a tour and got them settled in their bedroom.

I considered my in-laws to be good, decent people who were cautious about exhibiting their feelings. If they had thoughts or sentiments that they judged to be offensive to others, they hid them behind a facade of pleasantries. These "negative" emotions included sadness, anger, grief, and disappointment. During past visits with them, as a consequence, I had tended to dilute the intensity of my reactions to the world around me so as to spare them discomfort.

I had to admit that I was feeling nervous about their visit. I knew I did not have the wherewithal to be polite at all costs, or to withhold my feelings regarding Andrea. Tom and Edna would be seeing me vulnerable and defenseless. For my part, I would have to find the grace to accept them and their reactions (or lack of reaction) during this, the most sorrowful of times.

The four of us sat around the table eating and talking about The Farm, their trip to New York, the station wagon they had driven (and that Lowell and I were buying from them), and, of course, the weather. When I was first getting acquainted with Lowell's parents, I'd been struck by their propensity for discussing the weather, a subject I was wholly indifferent to. I soon learned that their preoccupation with the weather had much to do with the fact that Tom was a farmer and his livelihood depended on its cooperation. Also, the climate was a safe subject on which to comment, requiring no controversial observations. It was something, pretty much, that everyone could agree about.

Halfway through our meal Edna mentioned that Tom didn't really care for pizza. It was just like Tom not to complain or bother anyone with his preference. "I'm a meat and potatoes man," he said.

Naturally, we didn't talk about Andrea. Lowell had decided to tell them everything after dinner.

The next day, Lowell and his parents drove into Manhattan to see Andrea. I decided to stay at The Farm and commune with myself. I had just finished lunch when the phone rang.

"Hello, Mrs. Alecson?" a woman said.

"Yes."

"This is Dr. Laurel at the hospital. Your daughter, Andrea, has passed away."

"Andrea died?"

"Yes."

After a pause, I asked how she had died.

"Her heart stopped," Dr. Laurel answered.

"Thank God. Thank God, thank God . . . ," I chanted.

Immediately, I called our apartment to catch Lowell and his parents, hoping that they had stopped there before going to the hospital. No one answered, so I left a message for Lowell to call me as soon as he got in.

I then ran outside, dropped to my knees, and, raising my arms to the sky, continued to cry, "Thank God, thank God, thank God."

9

Grief and Renewal

I was seated cross-legged on the lawn vibrating with the news of Andrea's death when Lowell called.

"Lowell, a doctor from the hospital just phoned. Andrea died."

"My God, she did? How?"

"Her heart stopped."

"I can't believe it. Thank God." He started to cry.

After a few minutes I said, "We got what we've been asking for." Then I, too, started to cry.

"Are you coming into the city? Do you want to see her?" he asked.

I imagined driving to the train station, riding Metro North to Grand Central, then getting to the hospital by either subway or cab. Once I got there, I would not be able to be alone with her, and I would have Lowell's parents to consider and hospital personnel to contend with. I wanted to just feel my feelings, unbridled.

"Lowell, I need to be alone and meditate on all this without having to deal with anyone. I really don't feel the need to see her because I feel her presence all around me now. Is that okay? Can you go over there with your parents? Do you understand?"

"Of course I understand. I'm going to the hospital, and I'll call you from there. I love you."

"I love you, so much."

"Are you sure you'll be all right?" he asked.

"Yes."

I hung up the phone, poured myself some vodka, then walked around my parents' property with the glass in my hand. How ironic—if that was the word—that Andrea should die on the day her paternal grandparents were to see her for the first time.

The effusive emotions I was experiencing were similar to the ones I had had when I heard from Gloria that the ethics committee had decided to let Andrea die. I felt light-headed from a relief that knew no bounds, but my heart ached, and that dichotomy of sensation took possession of my body as I thought, "She is free, she is free, my baby is free."

I wandered around outside and talked to the heavens, pausing every so often, overcome by tears. The whole thing—her disastrous birth, the weeks of limbo, the resistance of West-One—all of it had been so unnecessary. All of it was so unfair. I was supposed to be celebrating the birth of my child, not her death.

I went back inside and called my mother, but there was no answer. Then Lowell called from the hospital.

"It's a good thing you didn't come," he said. "She doesn't look like herself. Her appearance has changed so much since we saw her the last time. She looks like a sleeping doll."

The doctor had asked if we wanted an autopsy to be done. I agreed with Lowell that we should request one. He sounded remarkably composed, considering what was happening. I recognized that his parents were a comfort to him.

"There's nothing left to do now, so we'll head back to The Farm," Lowell said after a pause.

"What should we do about dinner?" I asked, even as I thought, "What a normal thing to ask, especially since none of us will have an appetite."

"I don't know," he replied. We left it at that.

As I hung up the receiver I thought that it is precisely the mundane, the conformity of a schedule, that keeps us from being splintered apart by all that is out of our control. The ground could be shifting beneath our feet, but such daily indentations into the chaos of existence as breakfast, lunch, and dinner will prevent us from caving in, if we're lucky.

I had an hour before Lowell and my in-laws were to return. I put my sneakers on and ran along a flat stretch of road until I was exhausted. When they pulled into the driveway, they found me on the north side of the house, sitting on the stone rim of what used to be a silo, catching my breath.

Lowell walked over to me and we embraced, holding each other as his parents stood nearby. It wasn't dramatic, and we weren't hysterical. I then hugged Tom and Edna, noticing that Tom's eyes were red and swollen and that Edna was keeping it together as best as she could. She soon went about the business of dinner, unwrapping the fast-food hamburgers and french fries they had picked up en route.

The evening passed in somber disbelief. I called the number that Kitty had left, and the mortician who answered was indeed prepared to arrange everything. We asked that Andrea be cremated. We then took turns phoning a few of the people closest to us. My parents called from their inn; on hearing the news my father said, "I'm sorry, Deb. But this is what we've all wanted. It's for the best."

I reached my mother, and after she had stopped crying,

she wanted to know if we planned to have a service. I told her we didn't think so. "Lowell and I need to discuss it further, Mom."

Under the circumstances, a funeral didn't make sense to me. Funerals are for the living to say goodbye to the dead. They channel emotions into rituals that help give shape to grief. Funerals give you permission to lament, to feel remorse, to be under the spell of mortality. Lowell and I had been mourning the loss of Andrea, in our own ways, since she came into the world. For the two months of her suspended life, we had grieved.

Before going to bed I shared my thoughts with Lowell, but he said he needed more time to think about it.

I said, "I want to do something to acknowledge her and what we've been through, but I'm not sure what that is."

"We have time," he said. We held each other in the darkness for a while, then he went to talk with his parents.

I fell into a troubled sleep. In the middle of the night I was awakened by Lowell, who lay sobbing beside me.

The next morning, I realized that I should inform Ricky Pagan of Andrea's death. That meant tracking down his home number, since it was a Sunday and the law office was closed. I grappled with whether I should wait until Monday, but I felt an urgency, that he would want to know as soon as possible. I found his number listed in the Manhattan phone book, and he answered the phone.

"I apologize for disturbing you at home, but I thought you would want to know that Andrea has died."

To my astonishment, after the predictable consolatory remarks, he strongly suggested that this new development could alter everything. We were going from a "damaged baby case" to a "wrongful death case," he said, leaving me to surmise the significance of this shift. I presumed, because Andrea was only two months old, that her death would reap a lesser compensation for us—and a smaller fee for the lawyers.

We agreed to talk more during the week. After I got off of the phone I said to Lowell, "How naive of us to think that they actually cared about us, or about justice. I bet they drop our case."

"Deb, I'm not at all surprised. They want to make money."

The day passed in emotional waves of keeping myself in check around my in-laws and letting my feelings flow when alone on walks or in Lowell's presence. The gratitude that I felt toward fate, toward the great beyond for letting her die, was immense, but not vast enough to eclipse the sadness that inhabited my entire being. My parents were to return from their vacation on Monday afternoon, so Edna and I housecleaned, did laundry, and made sure that we kept ourselves occupied. I was impressed by the painstaking inspection she gave to the accumulated dust and filth on the staircases. While I went from bedroom to bedroom changing sheets and pillow cases, Edna could be found on her hands and knees extracting particles from the corners of each and every step.

Tom attended to the station wagon they had driven from Minnesota, which was now ours. From the pool, where I would take breaks from cleaning, I would watch Tom checking everything out as he changed the oil. It hadn't yet registered that Lowell and I had just purchased an automobile, a possession that would make our lives easier. We could have been given a brand new Mercedes Benz and I wouldn't have cared.

My parents' return escalated our collective busyness, as they unpacked, greeted the Allecksons, and got settled in the midst of an emotional climate of repressed sorrow. The focus of the evening was dinner, thank God, and Kitty officiated by delegating tasks: Edna was to husk the corn, I was to make the salad, and Lowell was to help my father set up the table and grill on the patio. Our efforts to keep things friendly, calm, and comfortable masked an inarticulate strain within each of us. Kitty drank more wine than usual, which made her talkative and theatrical compared to my in-laws, who spoke in a monotone, as Minnesotans are apt to do, using declarative statements which lacked any embellishment whatsoever. I, too, drank a lot considering how little I had eaten, and I slipped into an internal chamber, catching bits and pieces of conversation about the car, my parents' trip, The Farm, and farming in the Midwest. The cleanup after dinner was also a big production that kept us all engaged. As I cleared the table of dishes I became increasingly numbed by a lack of connection to my feelings.

The next morning, we packed the car, and Lowell and his parents drove to our apartment in the city. I stayed behind for a few hours to await a phone call from a car insurance company and to avoid Lowell's voice lessons. It was one of the hottest days of the summer thus far, and I stayed in a reclining position by the side of the pool.

I felt that the distractions of my in-laws' arrival and my parents' return had prevented me from fully absorbing Andrea's death. With the sun blazing all around, and the heat stupefying every living thing, I lay motionless with eyes closed.

Andrea's death was what I had been praying for, but it was a no-win situation. She would not go on and on for years as a mutilated soul, and for this I was thankful beyond words. But that it should have come to this, that she was not born whole and mine, was a disappointment I thought I would never get over.

This was the first bit of time I had had alone with my parents since their return. Before I caught the train to

Grand Central Station, my father and I talked. I had shown him two poems I had written about Andrea, and he now took that opportunity to tell me how impressed he was by the way I was handling things. "It's in times like these that a person's true character is revealed," he said.

We hugged each other, and it was awkward, as our hugs usually were. My father was proud of me because I wasn't blubbering all over the place. I was presenting a good front and sparing those around me—or, more specifically, sparing him. There weren't any times in my life, that I could recall, when my father had expressed pride in something I had done or in a way that I had behaved. It took the most horrible thing that could ever happen to bring out "the best" in me and prove to my father that I had character.

That afternoon, four days since Andrea died, I had a therapy appointment with Dr. Melner. I walked into his office and handed him a couple of photographs of Andrea taken in the NICU. He remarked, "I'm struck by how well defined her facial features are so soon after birth. Her essence is present."

"It's unbelievable that she's died. She could have lived for years," I said, wondering why I'd wanted Dr. Melner to see these pictures.

"Well," he said, still studying the photos, "her dying was something she did for you and Lowell, to pave the way for the next baby."

Dr. Melner had a knack for saying just the right thing. I started to cry, but soon abandoned my tears. Instead, I talked about the daily details of my life, how Lowell and I were dealing with her death, his parents, each other. I spoke matter-of-factly, as if I was giving a report entitled, "My Week after My Daughter Died."

Before ending our session, Dr. Melner referred to the continuation of therapy.

"I'm all right," I said. "I'm handling things. I'm even enjoying a few activities." I told him that we had tickets for a Broadway show that very night.

He was unimpressed. After a pause he looked at me and said, "I want to see you next week, to see just how great you're doing." The touch of sarcasm in his voice was effective. We made an appointment, and I walked out of his office feeling relieved that I would see him again.

I met Lowell for dinner at our local Chinese restaurant, where I gulped down the complimentary wine they poured so generously. We were to see *Shirley Valentine*, and the plan was for Edna to join us, and for Tom to stay home. Tom couldn't hear well enough to enjoy a live performance.

We were pressed for time, and Lowell left me to finish my meal while he went home to change clothes. As I left the restaurant, although I was still prepared to go to the show, I was feeling increasingly unstable. By the time I walked through the door of the apartment, I couldn't control myself. Without acknowledging Tom or Edna, who were sitting on the couch ready to greet me, I went directly to the bathroom and shut the door.

I began to sob and wail. I was aware that my lamentation was interfering with our plans, for it was only ten minutes till curtain. I could not stop crying; I managed, through the bathroom door, to tell Lowell that I needed to be alone and that Tom should take my place. Hunched over on the toilet seat, I heard Lowell explain, "She's upset and doesn't think she can enjoy the show, so why don't we just go?" I waited for them to leave before emerging. I got more wine and set up the typewriter with the intention of writing poems that would once and for all purge my soul and make me feel better.

For the two and a half hours that they were away, I got drunk. I had brief, incoherent phone conversations with a few people who called. My attempt to write meaningful poetry was hopeless anyway: I was too inebriated to make sense of my emotions or organize my thoughts. I called my mother, who listened as I repeated, "I've been holding all this in." My anguish could not be inhibited, and my mother stayed steady on the other end as I sobbed and heaved.

When Lowell and his parents returned after the show they found me sprawled on the carpet in the living room, dressed in a skimpy negligee, with candles lit, their flames sparkling in the darkness, and the music of Leonard Cohen blasting from the stereo speakers. They all stood in the doorway for a few seconds. I knew I was a shocking sight for my in-laws to behold. Edna said, "You look so pretty," then walked over and gave me a squeeze. She quickly retreated, and she and Tom turned to go upstairs (they had been staying in a neighbor's vacant apartment). "Good night, Deborah," Tom called as they closed the front door.

Lowell poured himself a glass of wine, stripped down to his underwear, and joined me on the floor. He held me as I continued to cry. Before passing out for the night, I recalled my session with Dr. Melner, his words echoing in my mind: "I want to see just how great you're doing."

I awoke with the first hangover I had had in years, but I felt lighter in spirit. I had survived a plunge into an abyss that I would necessarily return to again and again if I was to exorcise the anguish that was as tangible and as deep as the marrow in my bones. With Andrea's death came the end of my worries over what we would do with her as she grew older, and how we would go on with our lives. Those torments were replaced with mourning the loss of my daughter as I would have wanted her, alive and healthy. All I could do was feel my feelings (as my mother always advised), not be afraid of my pain, and have faith in the healing power of time.

My in-laws were to fly back to Minnesota on Saturday morning, and we all made a valiant effort to spend our last few days together with as little gloom as possible. We were waiting to hear from the funeral director, to claim Andrea's ashes. Ricky Pagan was to get back to us regarding the status of our case. And I began to read a book that brought me great solace.

Kathy Nolan had recommended *The Long Dying of Baby Andrew*, which finally arrived at my local bookstore. I started reading it the minute I got my hands on it. It was written by the mother and father of a premature baby, Andrew, who lived for six months in critical condition in a NICU. The book's style is that of journal entries kept by both parents during those six months; its content is deeply personal and emotionally searing. No words on a page, including those of *Playing God in the Nursery*, spoke to me as directly as Robert and Peggy Stinson's, as they tried in vain to take control of their son's life and death. In so many ways I identified with this couple: with what they went through, how they handled it, and what they thought and felt throughout. Peggy Stinson writes, "My own belief is that the use of heroic and experimental medical technology is often a moral outrage, showing callous disrespect for the sacredness of human life and pathetic inability to face the reality of human death. But how can I protect myself and my children from those who believe that terminating medical treatment, no matter what the circumstance, is murder?" (pp. 67–68). One day she admits, "I'm having trouble facing up to the simplest of daily routines. Like getting out of bed" (p. 69). And later, "What a ghastly position to force people into—having to fight publicly for the death of their own child" (p. 74). Finally, "Andrew is not our baby anymore—he's been taken over by a medical bureaucracy" (p. 115).

Their nightmare lasted four months longer than ours, and they also had a small daughter whose life was very much affected. I couldn't help but look ahead to learn if they went on to have another child. They did. Their son was born "without incident" about one and a half years after Andrew's death. Would Lowell and I be as fortunate?

Tom and Edna took us out to dinner Friday evening, the night before their departure, but first we treated them to drinks in a revolving restaurant at Times Square that displayed much of Manhattan aglow. From my window I looked upon a city peopled with many who have known greater sorrow than mine, as well as some who have yet to encounter a single disappointment. This is what I thought about as Edna, seated across from me, rambled on about the various sites that came into view. One small drink was enough to loosen her up, and she addressed her attention to the overwhelming backdrop of New York City, avoiding any discussion of Andrea.

Back at the apartment, before we were to retire for the evening, Edna brought out her camera and requested that we take turns posing on the couch. I was in no mood to plaster a smile across my face, but I reluctantly complied. Then, quite unexpectedly, while talking about how best to get to the airport, Edna and Tom began to cry.

"This has been a hard time for you guys," said Tom. "We sure hope things work out for you."

"We know it's for the best, how things worked out, but it's been a terrible thing," Edna said, putting her arm around my shoulders.

I was taken aback, unaccustomed as I was to such demonstrativeness from Lowell's parents. Tears welled in Lowell's eyes as he embraced his father. This was the most my in-laws had emoted since they'd arrived in New York, at least in my presence. I was so used to Edna's evasiveness and Tom's silence that this spontaneous and genuine show of feelings unnerved me.

"We'll be all right," I assured them.

"You've got each other," Tom said.

Once everyone's composure returned, we said goodnight.

While Lowell was with his parents at the airport, the funeral director called to say Andrea's remains were ready to be picked up. The place was a few blocks from the apartment, so I headed out, right after a morning swim, onto already steaming streets. I had no idea what to expect but imagined that I would receive a small vial filled with pearly-white powder. In the poorly lit parlor I found Sal, one of the undertakers, seated at a desk in the back office. Without formality, he handed me the certificates of death and cremation, together with a metal canister about the size of a small sack of flour.

I had thought that the claiming of the ashes would be traumatic. I suppose it would have been different if I had to see her dead but preserved, laid out in a coffin, her sweet little face before my eyes. That sight surely would have annihilated me. But this receptacle that I placed on top of the kitchen table was a foreign object to behold. Instead of eliciting tears, it made me wonder how a human life can be so reduced to rubble. Nine months of joyous expectation, a catastrophic birth that nearly killed me, and two months of battle with the powers that be to release my Andrea from a quasi-life . . . the whole experience had been transmuted into this tin cylinder that contained my answered and unanswered prayers. My child.

I decided to wait until Lowell and I were together before removing the lid. In the meantime, I studied the certificates and noted the statement, signed by the physician who pronounced her dead: "I further certify that traumatic injury or poisoning DID NOT play any part in causing death, and that death did not occur in any unusual manner and was due entirely to NATURAL CAUSES." I put the two documents in the folder with her birth certificate.

Lowell and I ran a few errands before opening the canister. As we sat side by side on the couch, I took off the cover. Inside we found a clear plastic bag fastened with a twistie; it contained quite a bit more ash than we'd anticipated. We cried softly and held each other.

"My God, there are actually little pieces of bone," Lowell said.

"I can't believe this is her," I replied.

We still didn't know what we would do with her remains, except to scatter them someplace that was special to us. I had a metal box painted with cheery flowers and a gold trimming that I had set aside when I was pregnant, thinking it would make a perfect holder for little cherished toys. We put her ashes in there and placed it on a shelf in the nursery.

In the mail, along with the goddamn bill from Dr. Henry for $341.00, was the postmortem record from the hospital's department of pathology. It was the final diagnosis and summary based on the autopsy. I didn't understand a word of it. What was clear, however, was that her brain was a mess and had been atrophying. A succinct diagnosis was written across the first page in capital letters: "SEVERE, DIFFUSE ANOXIC-ISCHEMIC ENCEPHALOPATHY AND LEUKOENCEPHALOPATHY." On the second page there appeared equally incomprehensible and terrifying descriptions. Using a dictionary, I translated some of the language and finally reached the simple and already known conclusion: a lack of oxygen had destroyed her brain, and bronchopneumonia had destroyed her lungs. If the latter condition could have been arrested with antibiotics, then maybe Dr. Kravitz used it as Andrea's way out.

That morning, I had gotten to the part in *The Long Dying of Baby Andrew* where the doctors finally agreed, unofficially, to let Andrew die. Peggy Stinson writes:

> Craft confirmed today what Farrell wouldn't admit—they took Andrew off the respirator so he could die, and now they're all waiting around for him to do it. Craft's "guess" is cardiac arrest, since Andrew can't breathe adequately enough without the respirator to prevent a really massive buildup of CO_2.
>
> They found their loophole. Because of course I shouldn't say they "took him off"—they couldn't do that, since that would be immoral and illegal. They had to hope for an appropriate accident; once Andrew became accidentally detached from the respirator and had breathed for a couple of minutes, they could declare him "off" and omit to put him back on while they wait for his inadequate breathing to kill him. This is the moral, legal, and "dignified" way. (p. 345)

Later, reflecting on his death, she writes, "Modern medicine makes possible a sad new epitaph: He died too late for grief" (p. 347). Andrea lived for six weeks after we had met with the specialists and beseeched them to let her die. Why we all had to endure those weeks, which could have been years or decades, is a question whose answer lies beyond the legal implications, real and imaginary, of withholding nutrition. Peggy Stinson would agree that Andrea was kept alive because of an individual and collective fear of death. I truly believed it was that simple, and I could only thank Dr. Kravitz for having the courage to take advantage of the "loophole" given to him.

"Lowell," I said as I handled Dr. Henry's bill, wondering

what to do with it, "I'm going to call the hospital and find out just who Dr. Henry is."

After being put on hold or transferred from one department to another, I finally found a woman in radiology who knew of Dr. Henry's existence. I started out calmly, "I'm calling because I've been receiving this bill, every single week it seems, from a Dr. Henry who claims to have done something for my daughter who was in the NICU. I never heard of him, and I never asked him to treat her."

"What is your daughter's name?"

"My daughter's name was Andrea Alecson. She died. And it's upsetting to get this bill in the mail addressed to her."

"Oh. I'm sorry."

I had to admit to a certain sadistic pleasure in telling this complete stranger, a woman who spent her days sending bills to disaster-stricken households, that my daughter was dead. She put me on hold as she scanned her computer for evidence of the bill.

"Mrs. Alecson," she began.

I interrupted, "Look, Andrea's stay at the hospital has cost tens of thousands of dollars. All we can do, my husband and I, is hope and pray our insurance company will cover most of it. With everything that was going on, we never got this bill to them, and now they claim it's too late to process. Certainly the hospital can live without our $341."

I was no longer listening to the woman as she attempted an explanation, saying, "Dr. Henry was a consultant for Dr. Maslin . . ."

I was clutching the receiver with all my strength. "I want to speak to Dr. Henry," I demanded.

"Well, I can leave him a message, but these consulting doctors do not have regular . . ."

"It's not fair," I yelled into the phone, "that we should be expected to pay for a doctor's service that we did not request. Would you tell Dr. Henry that our daughter has died, that we should not be responsible for that bill, and to leave us alone."

"I'll see what I can do. Maybe under these circumstances . . ."

I sensed that she was genuinely sympathetic, but I wouldn't acknowledge it. I said "Thank you," and hung up.

I knew, and Lowell knew, that I was venting a rage aimed at the hospital, and this poor woman, who was an innocent party, was simply doing her job. We could have just as easily viewed the $341 as a mere pittance compared to the final bill: a few hundred dollars that didn't greatly change the financial load. Instead, the money represented the powerlessness we had experienced all those weeks of Andrea's hospitalization. The call was an attempt to regain authority.

A yoga and meditation instructor at our health club with whom Lowell and I had taken a few classes, knowing of our tragedy, invited us to participate in a workshop the following morning. In sweat pants and T-shirts, we walked hand in hand to the club. I was feeling vulnerable, as usual. "Lowell," I said as we crossed the street, "I know it'll be good for us to do this together, but I'm a little nervous that I might fall apart."

"Jeffrey understands what we're going through, and I think he wants to help us, to give us the space to get in touch with our feelings."

"Yeah but, what if I lose it? What about the others?"

"Deb, honey, relax. This is for us. We can always leave."

I was having a hard time being in social settings; I had forgotten how to have conversations. While a yoga and meditation workshop was hardly a social occasion, it was an experience to be shared with others. The only thing that I had to share was my heartache. As Lowell and I entered the room, we received a gentle nod of welcome from Jeffrey. I looked at him, and our eyes locked for a moment. In that instant began a healing that continued throughout the morning. Lowell and I found spots next to each other on the carpeted floor, and no matter how far I journeyed within, I stayed ever aware of Lowell nearby, of our brave return to the light of the living.

That week, we decided to have a party instead of a funeral. We called our friends, old and new, including neighbors, women from the health club, nurses from the NICU, Jeffrey the yoga teacher, and some of Lowell's voice students. My parents were invited but would not come for reasons other than the usual one: my father's and mother's extreme discomfort when in the same room together. My father and stepmother were also anxious to disperse the cloud of Andrea that had been shadowing their lives. I imagined their position to be: Why continue her influence in everyone's life by having a sort of wake?

My mother was hurt that we had not considered her wish to have a formal service. Besides the fact that Lowell and I did not need such a service to feel a sense of closure, we were perplexed by the particulars. First of all, what does one conventionally do to memorialize the death of a baby whose brief life was an agony that no one wanted prolonged? If indeed we had a funeral, what kind would it be? My family on my mother's side is culturally Jewish, but not religious. Lowell's family is Lutheran, but he has no church affiliation. I didn't know what I believed in any more, except for the arbitrary blessings and misfortunes that befall believers and nonbelievers alike.

And who would attend a funeral? Most of Andrea's extended family was uninvolved. My sister had made one obligatory phone call when I was still in the hospital. Most of my cousins, while aware of what we were going through, hadn't contacted us while Andrea was alive, let alone sent cards of sympathy.

No—a funeral would not work.

The afternoon of the evening of our party, Ricky Pagan called to tell us that his firm would not be pursuing our case. He explained that as Andrea had died an infant, we would not procure much of a recovery because of "the value of life as defined by the state of New York."

He went on to say, "Our decision is not based on the validity of the case, the strength of the evidence indicating malpractice. You do have a strong case here. It's just that under the law, an infant's life is of little value."

"What does that mean?" I asked.

"Well, if you could get between twenty and thirty thousand, that would be a lot. And we feel it's not worth what the parents have to go through to obtain such a small amount. It hardly equals what she was to you and Lowell, her true value, and it doesn't make the reliving of it worthwhile. You know, these things can drag on for years."

I thought, "He's a lawyer; naturally thirty thousand dollars is small change to him." I said, "Thirty thousand dollars is a lot to me and Lowell. But of course you're right, no amount of money could replace Andrea."

"If Andrea had lived, there would have been enormous medical expenses to compensate for. It would have been a totally different situation. I'm sorry; maybe you'll want to find another firm, get another opinion. You know, we had a case of a newborn who died in his father's arms right after birth. There was clear negligence. That family went through hell, and you know what the courts awarded us? Twenty thousand dollars. Never again. It was too wrenching."

"Well, we're not surprised by your decision. We would like the records back, though, and we'll talk with Nancy and get her advice."

"I guess it's okay to have the records. Call me in a week or two and we'll arrange everything."

Lowell had overheard the conversation, and when I hung up he said, "I think they don't want to bother unless it's a million-dollar case."

I said, "What about justice? What about accountability? Kembel and June will continue to deliver babies, and I suppose no authority will check to see if they made a mistake. The whole situation is fucked up."

As we cleaned the apartment and prepared for the gathering, I thought about what I had learned from Pagan about the law's assessment of the value of life. He'd said something about a death being "a loss to the estate," and the criterion was the size of that loss. It was a little confusing, but the gist of it was that if, under the exact same circumstances, negligence caused the death of an employed father of two versus a retired widow, the recovery would be substantially greater for the father. The income that the dead person would have earned if he or she had lived was a deciding factor. Yet the retired widow would have put in many years as a contributing member of society. It didn't make sense. And what about potential life? Andrea had the potential, at least when she was in the womb, of growing up to be a wage earner and independent member of society. Didn't that count for something? Plus, the courts did not consider the emotional pain and suffering of the family. That was something, according to Pagan, that the courts would not attempt to measure. However, Andrea's pain and suffering could be measured—assuming it could be determined. Legally, if it was proven that she was in torture during those weeks as a result of the perinatal insult, the amount of recovery would increase. But not enough to satisfy Pagan, apparently.

I felt sick and angry at the way the system failed us. It

seemed that money was the issue, not a baby's lost life and her parents' grief.

The doorbell rang, and as I buzzed in friends I marveled at how I could possibly be so disappointed with the lawyers. It was as if I continued to cherish an idealism that was repeatedly shattered, no matter how many times I was let down by others.

Soon the party was in full swing, with Lowell at the piano and theater friends and voice students taking turns singing songs. It was as if they were each serenading the group. I had placed the multicolored box containing Andrea's ashes in a conspicuous place, beside one pink rose in a clear glass vase, and I circulated the two poems I had written. A couple of people asked to see a picture of Andrea, and I showed the only one I had of her, lying in my arms, tubes, wires, and all. That was the extent of my "ritual."

It was nearly midnight when Gloria arrived, having stopped at home to change into a dress after a twelve-hour shift at the NICU. We hadn't seen her for weeks, and I was overtaken with emotion when she entered the apartment. She, more than anyone else, had known Andrea. She had touched her, fed her, held her in her arms, changed her diapers, regulated her medications, given her sponge baths, and combed her hair. She was part of our family history. Tears filled my eyes as I settled Gloria into a chair. I felt such gratitude and love for this woman who, after a long day caring for sick newborns, made the effort to honor us and Andrea with her presence.

"Let me get you something. Would you like a glass of wine? Are you hungry? You must be tired. I'm so glad you came." And we hugged. There were tears in her eyes.

"I'm fine, really. I had dinner not too long ago."

"How about a little white wine?"

"Well, maybe a little. That would be nice."

As I scurried off to pour her a glass, I wished I had something to offer her that came close to equaling the thankfulness I felt for her kindness, for her very being.

With most of our guests departing, I was able to give my full attention to Gloria. We talked about her ailing mother and, of course, Andrea.

"She was very special to me. That's how it is. You work with babies all the time, and then there are a few you feel differently about. She was so beautiful. And I really wanted everything to turn out right for you guys. You've been through so much."

In bed, Lowell and I talked about the party.

"Did you know that Maria had only one child, who died at four months?" I asked. Maria the wife of José, the superintendent of the building.

"Really? With José?"

"I don't think so. With her first husband. I didn't get all the details; you know her English isn't great. Maybe it was crib death."

"How awful. Four months old."

I dissolved into sleep feeling blessed with friends and aware as ever that Lowell and I were hardly the only ones to have lived through loss.

That week, I finished the poem I had been working on about Andrea's death.

At Last You Are Free

No more calls to the NICU
asking about Baby Alecson.
In spite of those feedings
oozed down a tube
plunged in your newborn throat,
you had the strength
to die, making room
for another life.

I was vehicle
for a magical becoming
powered beyond me.
I understood yours
must be a separate destiny.
But your birth brought
attachments I couldn't control,
then questions whether you, alive,
were living at all.

I nurtured you inside,
sacred wonderment,
daughter of my dreams;
your fate was yours,
as mine is mine.

A few days later, my period arrived. I was waiting for that primordial event to begin a self-cleansing. I stopped drinking alcohol and caffeine, and prepared my body to be a friendly habitat for the seed of our next child.

Epilogue

In January 1990, I was at the Hastings Center doing research for what has turned out to be this book. I had been feeling ill for weeks, though after five months of trying to conceive I still wasn't pregnant. Concerned that Dr. Kembel, in the haste of my emergency Caesarean section, might have ruined my reproductive capacity, I had seen a fertility expert who did some tests. One morning, while working in the basement of the center, I received a call from the doctor's office that explained my physical discomfort. I was pregnant.

That September, our son, Skyler, was born, at the hospital where Andrea had died. He was delivered by the same obstetrician who, just weeks earlier, had delivered Nancy Cronin's son. Once again, my labor was difficult, and I had to have a Caesarean section. This time, though, I was awake during the procedure, and Lowell was by my side. Skyler, wide-eyed and alert, came into the world scoring an Apgar of ten.

One of my first visitors at the hospital, hours after the

birth, was Dr. Kravitz. No one could have been happier than he for this joyful end to a tragic ordeal.

Prior to my pregnancy, we had retained a lawyer to pursue our wrongful death suit. Nancy Cronin, feeling bad that Pagan and his firm had dropped our case, took it upon herself to find us an attorney. The lawyer, Joel Damsky, had great sympathy for what Lowell and I had endured. He recognized the possibility that malpractice could have occurred, and he believed in justice. Joel was also an older man who could afford to apply his expertise as an attorney to helping people, regardless of the size of the monetary compensation. During the months I was pregnant with Skyler, I spent many afternoons with this gentleman, piecing together Andrea's story. As it turned out, we were better rewarded for our efforts than Pagan and his firm had imagined possible. There was a settlement out of court. When I recently spoke with Joel, he reiterated that it was an "amicable settlement," and that June, Dr. Kembel, and the hospital did not admit liability.

We continued to be pestered by Dr. Henry's bill for $341, which in the end we reluctantly paid. We had no choice, for it was required that all outstanding medical bills be paid before the settlement money could be released.

I have been asked if I now discourage the use of midwives. I do not, though I did not use one to deliver Skyler. The terrible nightmare of Andrea's birth could have happened, and in fact did happen, with the involvement of an obstetrician. A great disappointment is that the competence of the midwife, June, and of Dr. Kembel will, I suppose, never be investigated. They will continue to deliver babies, their skills unexamined, as long as they have medical malpractice insurance. That is the way our society works.

I have also been asked if writing *Lost Lullaby* was painful to do. I have had periods of profound sadness and depression reliving it all. However, the act of remembering the details and, more importantly, the emotions has been self-healing. Most certainly, having Skyler made the evocation of that time easier. But in truth, *Lost Lullaby* is a story of affirmation. I did not go mad; my marriage not only stayed intact, it was strengthened; and I did not have to resort to killing my daughter. I not only survived my grief, but I found the joy I had so feared I had lost forever.

Had Andrea survived, Lowell's life and my life would have remained in suspension. I do not know if we would have gone on to have another child. I believe that my awareness of her presence in the world, a source of relentless heartache, would have destroyed me. I doubt *Lost Lullaby* would have ever been written.

Bearing witness by writing a book has converted my personal sorrow into our story, one among many. While my husband and I got what we wanted for our daughter—her release—the legal obstacles, both real and imagined, continue to traumatize families today.

That is why I wrote this book.

Family members are not the only ones traumatized. Even when allowing a baby to die is the most humane and medically appropriate alternative to keeping her alive, doctors, out of fear of legal retribution or social castigation, will choose to prolong life. Consequently, they are put in the position of being unable to do what they know to be in the best interest of their patients. This dilemma of conscience was experienced by Andrea's doctors; and our wish to have all treatment withdrawn, including her feedings through an IV and later a nasogastric tube, was thwarted by their dilemma.

Everyone's dilemma.

I do not view neonatology to be an evil, or doctors who keep profoundly damaged newborns alive to be demonic, though my experience with Andrea has made me wary of hospitals. There is no enemy here, just universal confusion over how to assess the appropriate use and the ultimate consequences of medical technology.

Premature infants who were once naturally aborted, condemned for whatever reason not to reach full term, are now being sustained by human ingenuity. Irreversibly brain-damaged infants who in the past might have died are now offered life. The wonder of it all—but for whom?

Then there are the individuals, mothers and fathers, husbands and wives, who become incapacitated because of illnesses, accidents, and the natural decline of the body. Who speaks for these people when tragic circumstances have made them unaware of their condition, unable to voice their needs, unknown to themselves and unrecognizing of the world around them? Who decides whether they are living or dying and what, if anything, must be done?

The issues of allowing someone to die and of who makes that decision when the person cannot do so himself (because of impairment or because that person is a baby) are central to Andrea's story. While I was writing this book the *New York Times* of May 12, 1992, ran the headline "New York Rule Compounds Dilemma Over Life Support." The article described how New York state law virtually precludes family members from making treatment decisions (such as whether to insert a feeding tube or to remove a respirator) for their hospitalized loved ones when these individuals have not prepared a living will or named a health-care proxy. Eighty-five percent of the American population has not prepared a living will. Only twenty-eight states acknowledge family members as surrogates in the absence of a living will. It was our misfortune to have had Andrea hospitalized in New York, one of the twenty-two other states.

In 1993, New York's governor Mario M. Cuomo put together a bill that would acknowledge the right of some family members and significant others to make such health-care decisions for incapacitated loved ones. The bill did not pass.

Andrea's brief existence has made me ever aware of the medical, ethical, and social issues that remain unresolved. These are and will increasingly be paramount concerns of the 1990s, and of the twenty-first century. At least five questions stand out.

First, what criteria should be used to determine whether a medical intervention is "ordinary" or "extraordinary" care? The elaborateness of the technology? The consequence of its use on a patient? In Andrea's case, the hospital considered forced feedings through a nasogastric tube to be ordinary care. To those of us who felt that hers was an existence that it would be cruel to preserve, that her natural process of dying was being thwarted by the feedings, it was extraordinary care. But why should this distinction make such a difference? Because it is the best way our society has, thus far, for grappling with the overwhelming power of medical technology. If we can divide the use of this technology into ordinary versus extraordinary care, we have at least two categories to help us define its appropriateness in any given case.

Second, who has the right to make decisions about treatment or nontreatment for an unconscious patient who has not left a living will, or for an infant or child: the family or friends closest to the patient, the doctors treating the patient, an ethics committee, hospital administrators, or the government? If Andrea had remained dependent on a respirator, our problem would have been to get the hospital to remove it. It is difficult indeed for doctors to stop what they have begun. Some people would judge removing a respirator to be "playing God"; yet these same people would not view using one in the first place as playing God. It is my conviction that the family should make treatment or non-treatment decisions, in consultation with the attending physicians and nurses. *Lost Lullaby* is my personal testimony in favor of the bill that was not passed in New York State.

Third, what constitutes living and what constitutes dying? Is breathing alone enough to determine whether someone is alive? Or is it important that one can also think? Is a respirating body a life that should be preserved, even without a functioning cerebral cortex? Had Andrea survived, with proper nutrition and hydration, antibiotics for infections (of which there would have been many), and good custodial care, she would have grown into a child and then, possibly, into an adult captive in a bed in an institution, eyes fixed open, mute, unable to move voluntarily. Aides would have had to turn her from side to side to prevent the festering of bedsores. Her limbs would have twitched and jerked from an ever-extending spasticity, and, on occasion, her entire body would have convulsed from seizures until stopped with massive doses of phenobarbital. She would have become increasingly unrecognizable as her facial features succumbed to swelling due to poor circulation. She would never have uttered a sound, except for reflexive cries in response to pain. Lacking control of her bladder and bowel, she would either have needed a catheter or been in diapers all her life. Infections would have continually plagued her: her body, weak and sluggish, would have been a breeding ground for parasites. She would have lain, day in and day out, week in and week out, year after year, with no awareness of herself as a human being or of her environment as the human world.

Everything and everyone would have been meaningless to her.

Is this living? Why did we have such a hard time stopping such an eventuality from happening?

Fourth, what criteria should determine whether or not a life should be prolonged? Should the quality of life be a factor? What about the cost, especially now, when a national goal is to prioritize health care? Who should carry the financial burden for the continued existence of irreversibly impaired persons? In the case of infants, is the exorbitant expense of a NICU stay cost-effective for babies who will never grow up to be productive citizens, loving sons or daughters, fulfilled adults? Finally, should the strength and resources of the family, and the availability of special social services, be determining criteria?

The final question that must be asked is, can death ever be welcomed? Or will individuals use medical technology to deny their own mortality, as well as that of their loved ones?

Western culture has lost sight of what is illness (which can be treated) and what is the natural deterioration of the body. The availability of medical procedures, drugs, organ transplants, and miraculous machinery that can buy us more time is interfering with what could be a most precious time of our lives: our dying. Medical technology is taking away a pinnacle experience of life. Instead of looking within ourselves for peace and wisdom and saying our goodbyes to the people who have meant most to us, we are frantic with fear, expecting and even demanding that our mortality be "cured." And those who most love us are robbed of the sacred time to come to terms with what will, inevitably, be a loss. Lowell and I were denied that time.

People feel that they not only owe it to themselves to live forever, but owe it to their families as well. To die, in our culture, is to be a failure; and to discuss the inevitability of dying is increasingly taboo. This lack of open dialogue and expressed feelings makes living in these modern times ever more inauthentic.

It is my hope that Andrea's story will make these intricate issues human, and will convince readers that death can and should be welcomed when the alternative is a living hell.

Selected Bibliography

There were a few books that I read during the time of Andrea that brought me solace, as well as pertinent information about the world of the NICU. Jeff Lyon, in his book *Playing God in the Nursery* (New York: W. W. Norton, 1985), explores the consequences of the federal laws that regulate and limit choices for both parents and doctors. He describes in detail the seemingly sadistic procedures that imperiled newborns endure as one operation after another is performed to keep them alive, often against the wishes of the parents and the better judgment of the doctors. Lyon covers the ethics of neonatal care and its cost-effectiveness, and projects into a future that includes surgery on fetuses while still in the womb.

The Long Dying of Baby Andrew by Robert and Peggy Stinson (Boston: Little, Brown, 1983) is composed of journal entries by both parents as they lived through the six months their critically ill, premature son was kept alive in an NICU. While reading the book I felt as if I knew the Stinsons, and that they, strangers whose voices rang true page after page, understood what Lowell and I were going through, what we thought and what we felt. I am pleased that I had the opportunity to thank Peggy Stinson personally for having given me, as well as countless other parents who have endured similar tragedies, her honest and uncensored experience, to which I could compare my own.

A book that brought me great comfort is Stephen Levine's *Who*

Dies? An Investigation of Conscious Living and Conscious Dying (New York: Anchor Press/Doubleday, 1982). It helped to remind me that we are, after all, mortal, and that Andrea's essence was not her damaged body, but her spirit, which lives on.

Those sections of *On Children and Death* (New York: Macmillan, 1983), by Elisabeth Kubler-Ross, that describe the fear of having more children after the death of a child were valuable to me. The book did not meet my needs completely because the parents discussed who had lost a child had wanted that child to live. My situation with Andrea was quite different in that respect. Yet Kubler-Ross has many worthwhile things to say about loss, acceptance, and going on with one's life: the psychological process of grieving.

I picked up a copy of *The Right To Die: Understanding Euthanasia* (New York: Harper & Row, 1986) by Derek Humphry and Ann Wickett at some point during the time we were fighting for Andrea's own right to die. While the book did not address our problems, it does present an argument in favor of mercy killing when requested by an individual, and it gives a historical perspective of this controversial subject.

While I was writing *Lost Lullaby*, two books were published that tell the stories of much-loved and wanted babies who died. The first, *Born Too Soon* (New York: Doubleday, 1991), by Elizabeth Mehren, resembles *Lost Lullaby* in that it is a first-person narrative, but unlike Andrea, Mehren's daughter, Emily, was born prematurely, and Mehren and her husband had hoped that she would survive. William Loizeaux, the father of a firstborn who suffered from a disorder known as VATER syndrome, writes an emotionally cathartic account of his daughter's brief life in a book entitled *Anna: A Daughter's Life* (New York: Arcade, 1993). Like the Stinsons' book, it consists of journal entries, but they are written in hindsight, beginning weeks after Anna's death.

Two books I can recommend that are academic in nature are *Which Babies Shall Live?: Humanistic Dimensions of the Care of Imperiled Newborns* (Clifton, N.J.: Humana Press, 1985), edited by Thomas H. Murray and Arthur L. Caplan; and Irving G. Leon's

When a Baby Dies: Psychotherapy for Pregnancy and Newborn Loss (New Haven, Conn.: Yale University Press, 1990).

Helen Harrison, a mother whose premature child was salvaged by medical technology and still survives with a multitude of impairments, has been a force behind the movement for family-centered neonatal care. Her book, *The Premature Baby Book: A Parent's Guide for Coping and Caring in the First Years* (New York: St. Martin's Press, 1983), is immensely informative for parents whose infants are in an NICU, premature or otherwise. Harrison has compiled a comprehensive list of resources, including parent support groups both for those whose babies are living and for those whose babies have died. Also listed are organizations for the disabled, useful books and articles, and a glossary of medical terms commonly used in an NICU. Harrison is also the author of numerous articles that focus on prematurity and its long-term effects, as well as the ethical issues involved in medical treatment of premature babies. I am in full support of the points she outlines in "The Principles for Family-centered Neonatal Care," *Pediatrics* 92, no. 5 (November 1993), an article that resulted from a conference she organized in June 1992, chaired by the editor of *Pediatrics*, called "Intensive Concern: Parents and Physicians Discuss Neonatology." Papers presented at this conference included personal testimony from parents, the results of research crucial to the debate on the use of medical technology for at-risk newborns, and arguments in favor of parental rights in the decision-making process. Helen Harrison can be contacted at 1144 Sterling Avenue, Berkeley, Calif. 94708.

Books that I have not read in their entirety but that I can suggest are *Born to Die? Deciding the Fate of Critically Ill Newborns* by E. Shelp (New York: Free Press, 1986); *Mixed Blessings: Intensive Care for Newborns* by J. Guillemin and L. Holmstrom (New York: Oxford University Press, 1986); and *A Time to Be Born, a Time to Die* by R. Gustaitis and E. Young (Reading, Mass.: Addison-Wesley, 1986).

Four of the most prominent journals that publish articles on the medical and ethical dimensions of life support for severely impaired newborns are *Pediatrics*, the *Hastings Center Report*, *Birth*, and the *New England Journal of Medicine*. They can be found in most public libraries.

Regarding Nancy Cruzan, I have been told by Christy Cruzan White (Nancy's sister) that Dr. Ron Cranford followed the case closely with articles and commentaries, some of which have been published in the *Hastings Center Report*.

Resources for Parents

While numerous organizations exist for parents with disabled children, specific to the condition or birth defect, there are virtually no organizations or support groups for parents who wish to stop life support for their hospitalized newborns. A parent whose baby is in an NICU must ask the social worker about relevant support groups. If the baby should survive, parents need to know whom to call regarding their options, which are basically three: home care, medical foster care, or institutionalization. Parents must be persistent to get information, for often the NICU staff is too busy to provide a comprehensive list of services (including phone numbers for Medicaid, SSI, and food stamps).

I can name three organizations sympathetic to the plight of parents who feel powerless to stop life support for their dying neonates:

Choice in Dying
200 Varick Street
New York, N.Y. 10014
1-800-989-9455

Choice in Dying provides counseling services for families.

The Nancy Cruzan Foundation
217 North Cass Street
Carterville, Mo. 64835
(417) 673-3735

This foundation offers information regarding the legal status of people in a persistent vegetative state (PVS), as well as support for family members having to make medical decisions for their loved ones.

> The Hastings Center
> 255 Elm Road
> Briarcliff Manor, N.Y. 10510
> (914) 762-8500

Personally, I am indebted to the Hastings Center for their help. A nonprofit organization that conducts research on ethical issues in medicine, it is also an humane place with knowledgeable staff members who can give information and guidance to parents.

Helen Harrison, in her book *The Premature Baby Book*, suggested these three organizations as well:

> Parent Care
> 9041 Colgate Street
> Indianapolis, Ind. 46268
> (317) 872-9913

> IVH [Intraventricular Hemorrhage] Parents
> P.O. Box 56-1111
> Miami, Fla. 33156
> (305) 232-0381

> The Pregnancy and Infant Loss Center
> 1421 East Wayzata Blvd., Suite 40
> Wayzata, Minn. 55391
> (612) 473-9372

Additional organizations that might be helpful:

> Children's Hospice International
> 901 N. Washington St., #700
> Alexandria, Va. 22314
> 1-800-242-4453

The above organization finds hospice care for terminally ill children, and provides financial support as well.

Adopt-A-Special-Kid-America (AASK)
6577 Mission St., Suite 601
San Francisco, Calif. 94105
1-800-232-2751

AASK locates and places children with special needs.

American Self-Help Clearinghouse
St. Clares–Riverside Medical Center
Denville, N.J. 07834
(201) 625-7101

This group helps families locate existing support organizations and offers assistance in starting a self-help group.

Compositor:	ComCom
Text:	11/14 Aster
Display:	Aster
Printer and Binder:	Haddon Craftsmen